Paediatric and Adolescent Gynaecology for the MRCOG

Paediatric and Adolescent Gynaecology for the MRCOG

Edited by

Naomi S. Crouch
St Michael's Hospital, Bristol

Cara E. Williams
Liverpool Women's Hospital

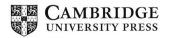
CAMBRIDGE
UNIVERSITY PRESS

CAMBRIDGE
UNIVERSITY PRESS

University Printing House, Cambridge CB2 8BS, United Kingdom

One Liberty Plaza, 20th Floor, New York, NY 10006, USA

477 Williamstown Road, Port Melbourne, VIC 3207, Australia

314–321, 3rd Floor, Plot 3, Splendor Forum, Jasola District Centre, New Delhi – 110025, India

103 Penang Road, #05–06/07, Visioncrest Commercial, Singapore 238467

Cambridge University Press is part of the University of Cambridge.

It furthers the University's mission by disseminating knowledge in the pursuit of education, learning, and research at the highest international levels of excellence.

www.cambridge.org
Information on this title: www.cambridge.org/9781108820769
DOI: 10.1017/9781108907507

First published 2023

Printed in the United Kingdom by TJ Books Limited, Padstow Cornwall

A catalogue record for this publication is available from the British Library.

Library of Congress Cataloging-in-Publication Data
Names: Crouch, Naomi S., editor. | Williams, Cara E., editor.
Title: Paediatric and adolescent gynaecology for the MRCOG / edited by Naomi S. Crouch, Cara E. Williams.
Description: Cambridge, United Kingdom ; New York, NY : Cambridge University Press, 2022. | Includes bibliographical references and index.
Identifiers: LCCN 2022022853 (print) | LCCN 2022022854 (ebook) | ISBN 9781108820769 (paperback) | ISBN 9781108907507 (ebook)
Subjects: MESH: Urogenital Diseases | Child | Adolescent
Classification: LCC RG110 (print) | LCC RG110 (ebook) | NLM WS 321 | DDC 618–dc23/eng/20220624
LC record available at https://lccn.loc.gov/2022022853
LC ebook record available at https://lccn.loc.gov/2022022854

ISBN 978-1-108-82076-9 Paperback

Contents

Contributors

Julie Alderson, DPsychol
Psychological Health Services, Bristol Royal Hospital for Children, Bristol, UK

Parivakkam S. Arunakumari, MD, FRCOG, MFFP
Department of Obstetrics and Gynaecology, Norfolk and Norwich University Hospital, Norwich, UK

Thomas R. Aust, MD, MRCOG
Wirral University Teaching Hospital NHS FT, Wirral, UK; Alder Hey Children's Hospital, Liverpool, UK

Adam H. Balen, MD, DSc, FRCOG
Leeds Teaching Hospitals NHS Trust, Leeds, UK

Katerina Bambang, PhD, MRCOG
Hewitt Centre for Reproductive Medicine, Liverpool Women's Hospital, Liverpool, UK

Joanne Blair, MRCP, MRCPCH, MD
Department of Paediatric Endocrinology, Alder Hey Children's Hospital, Liverpool, UK

Elizabeth Burt, MRCOG
Department of Obstetrics and Gynaecology, University College London Hospital, London, UK

Gail Busby, MRCOG
Division of Gynaecology, St Mary's Hospital, Manchester, UK

Matilde Calanchini, Md, PhD
Oxford Centre for Diabetes, Endocrinology and Metabolism, Churchill Hospital, Oxford, UK

Meenakshi K. Choudhary, MD, PhD, FRCOG
Newcastle Fertility Centre, International Centre for Life, Newcastle upon Tyne, UK

Samantha Cole, DPsychol
Psychological Health Services, St Michael's Hospital, Bristol, UK

Sarah M. Creighton, MD, FRCOG
Department of Women's Health, University College London Hospital, London, UK

Naomi S. Crouch, MD, MRCOG
Department of Gynaecology, St Michael's Hospital, Bristol, UK

Alfred Cutner, MD, FRCOG
Department of Women's Health, University College London Hospital, London, UK

Anju Goyal, FRCS(Paed)
Department of Paediatric Urology, Royal Manchester Children Hospital, Manchester, UK

Mugdha Kulkarni, MD, MRCOG
Leeds Fertility, Leeds Teaching Hospitals NHS Trust, Leeds, UK

Hazel I. Learner, MRCOG, MFSRH
Department of Women's Health, University College London Hospital, London, UK

Arianna Mariotto, MBBS
Department of Paediatric Urology, Royal Manchester Children's Hospital, Manchester, UK

Lina Michala, FRCOG, PhD
First Department of Obstetrics and Gynaecology, National and Kapodistrian University of Athens, Alexandra Hospital, Athens, Greece

Helen E. Turner, MA, MD, FRCP
Department of Endocrinology, Oxford Centre for Diabetes, Endocrinology and Metabolism, Churchill Hospital, Oxford, UK

Cara E. Williams, MRCOG
Alder Hey Children's Hospital and Liverpool Women's Hospital, Liverpool, UK

Ephia Yasmin, MD, MRCOG
Department of Women's Health, University College London Hospital, London, UK

Introduction

Paediatric and adolescent gynaecology (PAG) is a subspecialty that encompasses a broad spectrum of conditions affecting girls from birth up to adulthood. For younger children, vulval dermatological conditions are frequently seen, whilst the adolescent population will often present with menstrual dysfunction or pelvic pain, with a range of aetiologies. Rarer conditions, such as disorders of puberty, including precocious puberty, delayed puberty and primary amenorrhoea, may be associated with complex underlying conditions and are therefore appropriately managed in conjunction with paediatric endocrinologists. The more rare congenital gynaecological anomalies, including differences in sex development and Müllerian duct anomalies, will often present initially at adolescence to a local gynaecology service but are more complex and require specialist multidisciplinary team input in tertiary centres.

This book is aimed at trainees in gynaecology and reproductive medicine and consultants with an interest in PAG. It also provides detailed guidance and knowledge for all health care professionals working in the multidisciplinary team providing care for girls with gynaecological conditions, providing practical information about appropriate management and when to refer on.

Chapters 1–6 cover normal embryological development and puberty, history taking and examination and the more common PAG conditions. Chapters 7–15 cover the more complex conditions, including safeguarding and legal aspects of PAG. Key learning points are highlighted at the end of each chapter.

We have been delighted to work with authors within the field of PAG who have been selected as international experts in their fields and hope this book will inform and inspire future generations of PAG clinicians.

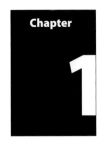

Embryological Development of the Internal and External Female Genitalia

Arianna Mariotto and Anju Goyal

The development of internal and external genitalia starts from the same baseline embryological point. From the ninth week of gestation, it diverges to differentiate into either male or female, depending on chromosomes, genes and hormones. The development of internal female genitalia is closely linked to that of the urinary tract; hence relevant details of urinary tract embryology will be outlined in this chapter.

1.1 Control of Sex Differentiation and Genetics

In species with heteromorphic sex chromosomes, such as human beings, sex differences arise from the genetic differences found in the sex chromosomes. The numerous sex-specific and sex-biased factors that interact in the network of genes and molecules and result in sexual differentiation are called *sexome* [1]. Female-biasing factors include two X chromosomes, ovarian hormones; male-biasing factors include a single X chromosome, the Y chromosome, and testicular hormones. The primary sex-determining factors are encoded by the sex chromosomes and are the only factors that differ in the male and female zygote. The secondary factors involve genes that are coded in the autosomal chromosomes [1,2].

The key role in sex differentiation in male development is played by *SRY* (sex-determining region on Y chromosome), a transcription factor derived from the short arm of the Y chromosome (Yp11). *SRY* initiates a cascade of downstream genes that determine the male development. It acts directly on the gonadal ridge and indirectly on the mesonephric duct for the development of the testes. It also causes the activation of genes that inhibit ovarian differentiation, and it upregulates steroidogenesis factor 1 (SF1), which through the SOX9 gene causes the differentiation of Sertoli and Leydig cells [3,4].

Absence of *SRY* in conjunction with positive mediation by specific genes on X chromosome causes the zygote to develop into a female. The X-linked and autosomal genes initiate ovarian development and block testicular differentiation. The two main genes involved in female sexual differentiation are DAX1 and WNT4. DAX1 is a member of the nuclear hormone receptor family located on the short arm of the X chromosome and acts by downregulating SF1 activity. WNT4 is a growth factor early expressed in the genital ridge that is maintained only in females and contributes to ovarian differentiation [2,3,5].

In addition to genes, sexual differentiation is affected by the hormonal milieu of the developing baby and end receptor sensitivity to hormones. Abnormal hormonal production by the placenta or adrenal cortex, or extraneous hormonal influence, or receptor insensitivity to hormones can affect sexual development, which may be contrary to that which would be expected from genetic sex.

1.2 Stages of Sex Differentiation

1.2.1 Early Development of the Zygote

Organogenesis occurs in the first 10 weeks of gestation and the remaining 28 weeks are spent in maturation, growth and development of function.

After fertilisation, the developing zygote divides and forms the blastocyst (Figure 1.1a). Later, two cavities – the amniotic cavity and the yolk sac – develop. The embryo arises from two layers of cells interposed between these two cavities, ectoderm and endoderm (Figure 1.1b). At approximately 15 days, an ingrowth of cells from the primitive streak forms a third layer between them, the mesoderm (Figure 1.1c). At the head and tail ends of the embryo, the mesoderm is deficient, resulting in the development of the buccopharyngeal and the cloacal membrane, respectively. The mesoderm is divided into three parts: lateral plate mesoderm, intermediate mesoderm and paraxial mesoderm (Figures 1.1d and 1.2a). Gonads, kidneys and genital ducts develop from the urogenital ridge on the

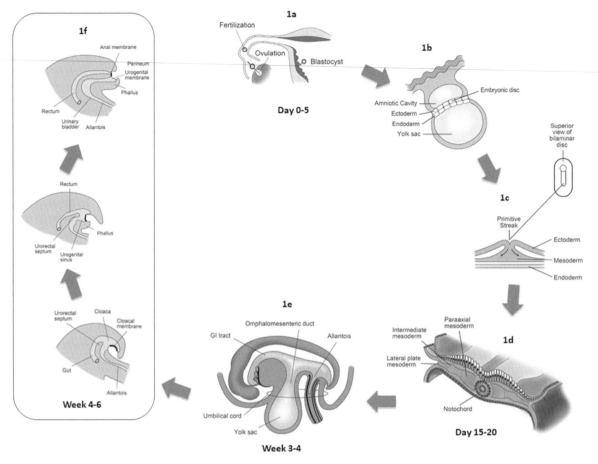

Figure 1.1 Early zygote development. (a) From fertilisation to implantation, first 5–6 days. (b) Development of two cavities – the amniotic cavity and the yolk sac – and bilaminar embryonic disc: endoderm and ectoderm. (c) Formation of third layer (mesoderm) from primitive streak. (d) Differentiation of mesoderm into paraxial, intermediate and lateral plate mesoderm. (e) Cephalocaudal folding of the embryo and development of early bladder (allantois), defining cloaca as part of hindgut distal to allantois. (f) Division of cloaca into urogenital sinus and anorectal canal by urorectal septum.

intermediate mesoderm (Figure 1.2b). Definitive kidneys develop from the nephrogenic cord (Figure 1.2c), which is divided craniocaudally into pronephros (primitive kidney – disappears)/mesonephros (intermediate kidney – disappears)/metanephros (definitive kidney). Two symmetrical pairs of genital ducts – mesonephric (Wolffian) and paramesonephric (Müllerian) ducts – develop lateral to the nephric blastema (or nephrogenic cord) (Figure 1.2c) and give rise to internal male and female genitalia. Gonads develop anteromedial to the mesonephros, from the genital ridges (Figure 1.2c).

Between the third and fourth weeks of gestation, head and tail ends of the embryo fold cephalocaudally. The endoderm of the yolk sac is included within the two folds and forms the gut. The allantois gains continuity with the developing gut and delimits the cloaca as the

portion of hindgut distal to their confluence (Figure 1.1e). Between the fourth and sixth weeks of gestation, the cloaca is subdivided into the primitive urogenital sinus anteriorly and the anorectal canal posteriorly by the descent of the urorectal septum, from the point of confluence of allantois and hindgut, towards the cloacal membrane/perineum and laterally by the folds of Rathke (Figure 1.1f) [3,6,7].

1.2.2 Development of Gonads

Gonads appear as a pair of longitudinal ridges (**genital** or **gonadal ridges**) sited on the anteromedial aspect of the mesonephros, the intermediate kidney (Figure 1.2c). Derived from intermediate mesoderm and overlying epithelium, these ridges initially do not contain germ cells.

During the third week of gestation, primordial germ cells appear on the wall of the yolk sac close to the allantois. Subsequently, they migrate along the dorsal mesentery of the hindgut (Figures 1.2d and 1.2e) to the primitive gonads (fifth week). During the migration they proliferate through mitosis and in the sixth week they invade the genital ridges (Figures 1.2d and 1.2e). Throughout this period, the epithelial cells of the genital ridge proliferate and penetrate the underlying mesenchyme, forming the **primitive sex cords**. At this stage, the gonad is undifferentiated (Figure 1.2e). The primitive sex cords and the primordial germ cells are found in both the cortical and the medullary zone and it is not possible to distinguish between male and female gonads. The initial formation of the bipotential gonad requires two transcription factors: Wilms' tumour 1 (WT1) and SF1. *SRY* is pivotal in further sexual determination and interplays mainly with two genes: SOX9 and DAX1, determining the differentiation into testis or ovary.

Due to their inductive influence on the development of gonad into ovary or testis, if the germ cells fail to reach the ridges, the gonads do not differentiate. From the sixth week, differentiation of gonads into testis or ovary occurs. In XX embryos the ovary will originate from the cortex and medulla will decline. In the XY embryo, medulla will develop into testis and cortex regresses [3,6–8].

1.2.2.1 Ovary

The ovary develops later than the testis and until the tenth to eleventh week, it does not have distinguishable histological features.

Once primordial germ cells have arrived in the gonad of a genetic female, they differentiate into **oogonia** and undergo several mitotic divisions (Figures 1.2e and 1.2f). In the meantime, in the presence of XX chromosomes and absence of *SRY* gene, the primitive sex cords degenerate. Instead, the epithelium of the gonad continues to proliferate producing secondary sex cords called **cortical cords**, that extend from the surface epithelium. As these cords increase in size, the primordial germ cells are incorporated into them. In females, the secondary sex cords retain their connection to surface epithelium and, therefore, the primordial germ cells are mainly found in the cortex (Figures 1.2e and 1.2f). Only a few of the sex cords reach the medulla, but those that go into depths and lose contact with the coelomic epithelium tend to undergo atrophy.

Oogonia proliferate by mitosis and then enter the first prophase of meiotic division to form **primary oocytes**. By the end of the third month of gestation, the oogonia are surrounded by a single layer of flattened epithelial cells which constitute the supporting cell lineage (**granulosa** or **follicular cells**) and are arranged in clusters (Figure 1.2g). By the fifth month of prenatal development, the total number of germ cells in the ovary reaches its maximum at about 7 million. However, many germ cells are lost during development. By the seventh month, all the surviving germ cells have entered meiosis and further germ cell development is arrested until puberty. A primary oocyte, together with its surrounding flat epithelial cells, is known as **primordial follicle**. The number of primordial follicles at birth amount to between 300,000 and 2 million, decreasing to 40,000 at puberty. Only about 300 primary oocytes develop further between puberty and menopause into fertilisable oocytes [3,7,8].

1.2.2.2 Developmental Anomalies

Turner syndrome is a chromosomal condition that affects ovarian development in females. It can be caused either by monosomy X or by X chromosome mosaicism and results in early loss of ovarian function (ovarian hypofunction or premature ovarian insufficiency) due to premature death of oocytes and degeneration of ovarian tissue. Many affected girls do not undergo puberty unless they receive hormone therapy, and most have significantly reduced fertility [7,8].

1.2.2.3 Testis

The testis develops earlier than the ovary. In the presence of XY chromosome complex, the *SRY* encodes for the testis-determining factor (TDF) and regulates the proliferation of the primitive sex cords and their penetration into the medulla to form the testis. A part of these cords forms the future rete testis and the other part containing germ cells and Sertoli cells becomes seminiferous tubules. The Leydig cells, located between the cords, start producing testosterone from the eighth week, driving the differentiation of internal and external genitalia [6,7].

1.2.3 Differentiation of Internal Genital Organs and Ducts

1.2.3.1 Molecular Regulation of Genital Duct Development

The male and female genital tract is undifferentiated until the ninth week of development. The mesonephric

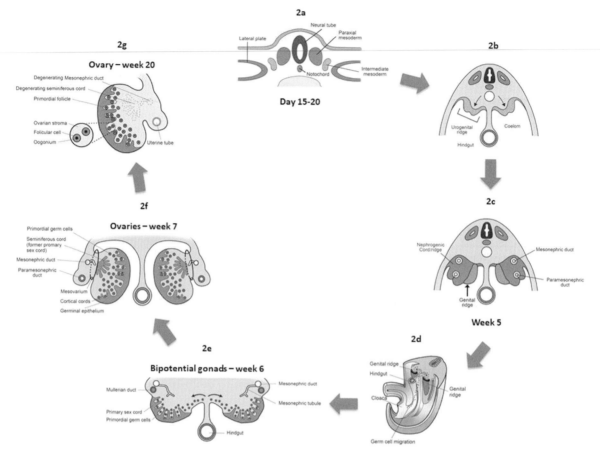

Figure 1.2 Gonadal development. (a, b) Cross section of the embryo showing intermediate mesoderm, which gives rise to the urogenital ridge. (c) Urogenital ridge differentiating into nephrogenic cord laterally and genital ridge medially. (d) Longitudinal section of the embryo showing migration of primordial germ cells into the genital ridge, from the yolk sac along the wall of the hindgut and the dorsal mesentery. (e) Cross section showing germ cell penetration into the genital ridges. (f) Early phase of ovarian development. (g) Advanced phase of ovarian development with degeneration of mesonephric duct.

and paramesonephric ducts together with the urogenital sinus give origin to the internal genitalia.

Female sexual differentiation, hitherto thought to be a default mechanism that occurs in the absence of a Y chromosome, is an active process mediated by specific genes on X chromosome. **DAX1** downregulates the SF1 activity, preventing the differentiation of Sertoli and Leydig cells in gonads. The growth factor **WNT4** contributes to ovarian differentiation. In the absence of MIS (Müllerian inhibiting substance, also called anti-Müllerian hormone/AMH), the paramesonephric ducts are stimulated by oestrogens to form the fallopian tubes, uterus, cervix and upper vagina. Oestrogens also act on the external genitalia.

In male embryos, *SRY* induces testicular development and differentiation of Sertoli and Leydig cells.

They produce MIS and testosterone, respectively. AMH causes regression of the paramesonephric ducts, while testosterone and its derivative dihydrotestosterone (DHT) mediates development of the mesonephric ducts into epididymis, rete testis, vas deferens, ejaculatory ducts and seminal vesicles. It also induces differentiation of the male external genitalia [3,5,7].

1.2.3.2 Genital Duct Differentiation

The paramesonephric duct emerges as a longitudinal invagination of the epithelium on the anterolateral surface of the urogenital ridge (Figure 1.3a). Cranially, the duct opens into the abdominal cavity with a funnel-shaped structure (abdominal ostium of the fallopian tubes) and it runs lateral to the mesonephric duct.

Caudally, it crosses ventrally and towards the midline, coming in close contact with the paramesonephric duct from the opposite side. The two ducts meet and fuse in a Y shape, forming the **utero-vaginal duct** (Figure 1.3b). Initially the two ducts are separated by a septum, but later on this vanishes and forms the uterine canal (ninth week). The point of contact of the Müllerian ducts with the urogenital sinus is called Müllerian tubercle (Figure 1.3b). The mesonephric ducts open into the urogenital sinus on either side of the Müllerian tubercle and later regress in the female (Figure 1.3c).

After the ducts fuse distally in the midline, a broad transverse peritoneal fold is established. This fold, which extends from the lateral sides of the fused paramesonephric ducts towards the wall of the pelvis, is the **broad ligament of the uterus**. The fallopian tube lies in its upper border and the ovary lies on its posterior surface. The uterus and broad ligaments divide the pelvic cavity into an anterior and a posterior pouch, respectively the uterovesical and the uterorectal pouch. Remnants of the mesonephric ducts are common in the broad ligament (Figure 1.3f).

The fused paramesonephric ducts give rise to the corpus and cervix of the uterus (Figures 1.3d and 1.3e). They are surrounded by a layer of mesenchyme that forms the muscular wall of the uterus, the myometrium, and its peritoneal covering, the perimetrium [9,10].

The vagina has a dual origin, the upper two-thirds derive from the paramesonephric ducts, whereas the

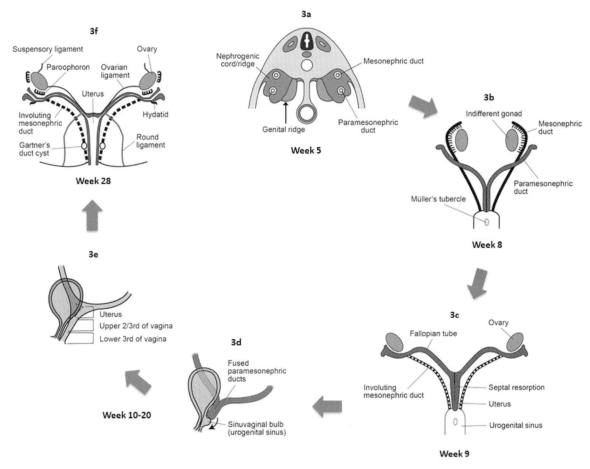

Figure 1.3 Paramesonephric duct development. (a) Paramesonephric duct arising as invagination of peritoneum over the nephrogenic ridge. (b) Distal part of paramesonephric ducts join in the midline. (c) The unfused part of paramesonephric ducts forms the fallopian tubes; the distal fused part gives rise to the uterus and the upper two-thirds of the vagina. (d, e) Development of the vagina from distal fused paramesonephric ducts and urogenital sinus. (f) Regression of mesonephric ducts with embryonic remnants proximally and distally. Peritoneal fold forming the ovarian ligament and round ligament of the uterus.

lower third derives from the urogenital sinus (Figure 1.3e). Shortly after the paramesonephric ducts reach the urogenital sinus, two solid evaginations grow out from its posterior wall creating the **sinovaginal bulbs** (Figure 1.3d). These proliferate and form a **solid vaginal plate,** which elongates and canalises by the twentieth week, giving rise to the lower third of the vagina. Between the third and fifth months, proliferation continues at the cranial end of the plate, increasing the distance between the uterus and the definitive vestibule (Figure 1.3e). The lumens of the vagina and of the definitive urogenital sinus are separated by a thin tissue plate which will partially degenerate after the fifth month. Its remnant, the hymen, consists of the epithelial lining of the sinus and a thin layer of vaginal cells. During perinatal life it develops a small opening. If this fails, an **imperforate hymen or variations thereof, such as septate or microperforate**, can develop. The urogenital sinus caudal to the vaginal opening becomes the **vestibule** [3,7,11,12].

1.2.3.3 Uterine and Vaginal Developmental Anomalies

Incomplete fusion of the Müllerian ducts gives rise to a variety of uterine and vaginal anomalies depending on the level of the anatomical defect, whether limited or throughout the entire line of fusion.

Uterus didelphys develops from complete failure of fusion of the paramesonephric ducts, partial failure results in **bicornuate uterus** or **arcuate** uterus. The lack of fusion of the two sinovaginal bulbs causes development of a **double vagina**. In contrast, **lower vaginal atresia** occurs if the bulbs do not develop at all. In this case a small vaginal pouch derived from the caudal part of the paramesonephric ducts surrounds the opening of the cervix. Defect in canalisation causes **transverse vaginal septa** and **atretic** segments of vagina.

Mayer–Rokitansky–Küster–Hauser (MRKH) **syndrome** is a rare disorder characterised by incomplete development of the Müllerian duct. It results in failure of uterus and vagina maturation and these may be atretic or absent. Women with this condition have normal ovarian function and external genitalia. They develop normal secondary sexual characteristics during puberty, but have primary amenorrhea.

Vestigial remnants of the mesonephric ducts may remain at proximal and distal ends and are usually found in broad ligament and adjacent to vagina. They are the epoophoron and paroophoron and the duct of

Gartner in the wall of the vagina (Figure 1.3f). These can undergo cystic malformation later in life resulting in **paraovarian cysts** and **Gartner cysts** [7,11,12].

1.2.3.4 Descent of the Ovaries

Gonads, together with the kidneys, develop retroperitoneally. During fetal growth, both female and male gonads undergo anatomical descent, the ovaries moving into the pelvis and the testes into the scrotal sacs. Descent of gonads is considerably less in the female than in the male, as the ovaries finally settle just below the rim of the true pelvis. Similar to males, a gubernaculum-like structure develops and extends from the inferior pole of the ovary to the subcutaneous fascia of the presumptive labioscrotal folds. It penetrates the abdominal wall through the inguinal canal and carries a slip of peritoneum with it called processus vaginalis. Although the gubernaculum does not shorten like that in males, it still causes the ovaries to descend (by anchoring the ovaries in the pelvis) and places them into a peritoneal fold (the broad ligament of the uterus). This translocation of ovaries occurs during the seventh week, when the gubernaculum becomes attached to the developing Müllerian ducts. The inferior part of the gubernaculum becomes the **round ligament of the uterus** and attaches the fascia of the labia majora to the uterus. The superior part of it becomes the **ligament of the ovary**, connecting it to the uterus (Figure 1.3f). As in males, the processus vaginalis of the inguinal canal is usually obliterated, but occasionally it remains patent and can result in an indirect inguinal hernia or hydrocele [3].

1.2.3.5 Differentiation of External Genitalia

External genitalia development occurs in two stages: hormone-independent growth and hormone-dependent growth.

1.2.3.5.1 Hormone-Independent Growth

This first phase of the development occurs between conception and the seventh to eighth weeks of gestation. It is similar in both genders as the external genitalia are undifferentiated until the ninth week.

This stage is influenced by a cascade of genes including sonic hedgehog (SHH), MNP4, Glia 123 and WT1 gene.

Around the third week, mesenchyme cells migrate from the region of the primitive streak to the perineum, around the cloacal membrane, to form elevated **cloacal**

folds on each side. Anterior to the opening of the urogenital sinus, cloacal folds fuse in midline to form the **genital tubercle**, which later develops into clitoris in females. At the sixth week, cloacal folds are subdivided into **urethral folds** anteriorly and **anal folds** posteriorly (Figure 1.4a).

In the meantime, lateral to the urethral folds, a pair of larger swellings – the **labioscrotal folds** or **genital swellings** – become apparent (Figure 1.4b). These join posteriorly, between the urogenital and anal membranes as they separate. The labioscrotal folds later form the labia majora in females and the scrotal sacs in males [3,4,6,7].

1.2.3.5.2 Hormone-Dependent Growth: Female

Sexual differentiation of external genitalia is hormone-dependent in both sexes. The development of external genitalia is determined by the hormones produced by the gonads, the correct steroid metabolising enzymes pool and the functioning sex hormones receptors. Impairment of any of these factors or environmental influences can cause alterations in the normal pathway.

Female differentiation of the external genitalia begins by the eleventh week and genitalia are defined by the twentieth week of gestation. In female fetuses, oestrogens stimulate the development of the external genitalia:

- The genital tubercle elongates only slightly and the phallus bends inferiorly forming the clitoris.
- The urethral folds remain unfused and develop into the labia minora.
- The genital swellings enlarge and form the labia majora.
- The urogenital groove remains open and forms the vestibule in which the urethral meatus, the vaginal orifice and the ostium of the vestibular glands are located (Figure 1.4c).

In addition to oestrogens, the development of external genitalia is promoted by the absence of androgens (dihydrotestosterone). All oestrogens are synthesised from androgen precursors by a unique enzyme called aromatase. Aromatase converts androstenedione, testosterone and 16-hydroxytestosterone into oestrone, oestradiol and oestriol, respectively. Defects in the

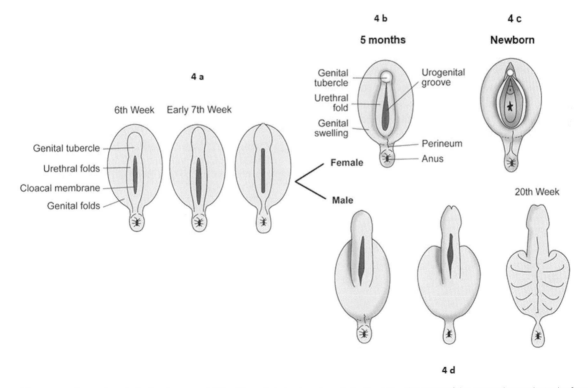

Figure 1.4 External genitalia development. (a) Undifferentiated external genitalia. (b, c) Development of the external genitalia in the female with appearance at 5 months and in the newborn, respectively. (d) Development of the external genitalia in the male.

aromatase gene result in elevated testosterone and virilisation. Other common causes of exposure to androgen include **congenital adrenal hyperplasia** (CAH). In the process of virilisation, there is trend towards elongation of genital tubercle (enlarged clitoris), fusion of labia majora (scrotalisation of labioscrotal folds) and fusion of urethral folds (urogenital sinus formation) [3,5,7,9].

1.2.3.6 Embryology and Congenital Anomalies

A good understanding of the embryological development of ovaries, internal and external genitalia will help a clinician in the assessment of anatomical anomalies that can result from a difference in expected development. An improved comprehension of developmental anomalies is a prelude to correct management planning and treatment.

Key Learning Points

- The development of internal and external genitalia starts from the same baseline embryological point, and it diverges after the ninth week of gestation into either male or female, depending on the influence of chromosomes, genes and hormones.
- Primordial germ cells migrate from the yolk sac to the genital ridges starting at the fifth week of gestation, forming the primitive undifferentiated gonads.
- After the tenth week, in the female, the primordial germ cells become primary oocytes and, together with the surrounding epithelium, form the primordial follicle. At this stage the gonad is differentiated into ovary.
- From the ninth week of gestation, the absence of anti-Müllerian hormone and the effect of oestrogens released by the ovary cause the differentiation of the paramesonephric ducts into fallopian tubes proximally, uterus, cervix and upper vagina distally.

- The external genitalia differentiation is mediated by oestrogens and absence of androgens in female and androgens in males.

References

1. Arnold AP, Lusis AJ. Understanding the sexome: measuring and reporting sex differences in gene systems. Endocrinology. 2012;**153**(6):2551–5.

2. Arnold AP, Chen X, Itoh Y. What a difference an X or Y makes: sex chromosomes, gene dose, and epigenetics in sexual differentiation. Handb Exp Pharmacol. 2012;(**214**):67–88.

3. Larsen WJ. Human embryology. 3rd ed. New York: Elsevier; 2002.

4. Catherine R, Rien N. Congenital anomalies in children. Vancouver, ON: SIU-ICUD; 2013.

5. Blaschko SD, Cunha GR, Baskin LS. Molecular mechanisms of external genitalia development. Differ Res Biol Divers. 2012;**84**(3):261–8.

6. Gearhart J, Rink R, Mouriquand P. Pediatric urology. 2nd ed. Philadelphia: Saunders; 2009.

7. Thomas D, Duffy PG, Rickwood AMK. Essentials of paediatric urology. 2nd ed. Scottsdale, AZ: Informa; 2008.

8. Makiyan Z. Studies of gonadal sex differentiation. Organogenesis. 2016;**12**(1):42–51.

9. Sajjad Y. Development of the genital ducts and external genitalia in the early human embryo. J Obstet Gynaecol Res. 2010;**36**(5):929–37.

10. Robboy SJ, Kurita T, Baskin L, Cunha GR. New insights into human female reproductive tract development. Differ Res Biol Divers. 2017;**97**:9–22.

11. Cunha GR, Robboy SJ, Kurita T, Isaacson D, Shen J, Cao M, et al. Development of the human female reproductive tract. Differ Res Biol Divers. 2018;**103**:46–65.

12. Walsh PC, Retik AB, Vaughan EB, Wein AJ. Campbell's textbook of urology. 12th ed. Hoboken, NJ: Elsevier; 2020.

Gynaecological History and Examination in Children and Adolescents

Hazel I. Learner and Sarah M. Creighton

2.1 Introduction

This chapter discusses the history and examination of children and young people with gynaecological concerns. A child refers to a younger child who lacks the understanding or maturity to make important decisions for themselves. Older and more experienced children (generally adolescents) who can make these decisions are referred to as young people [1].

A Paediatric or Adolescent Gynaecology (PAG) consultation may be fraught with anxieties.

- The transition through puberty is varied, and changes may be mistaken as signs of disease rather than a normal manifestation of pubertal development.
- A parent's or caregiver's experience of gynaecological review will typically have included speculum examinations; many people assume an internal examination a standard part of a gynaecological review.
- The gynaecologist may feel apprehension – they may have not seen many children and young people. They may have limited experience in the condition or co-morbidity that has prompted the PAG referral.

An unsatisfactory experience with a gynaecologist as a child or young person can impact on their long-term health. For instance they may be more reluctant to attend for sexual health advice or to engage with the cervical screening programme.

2.2 The Setting

Acute PAG reviews should be seen in the children's emergency department. Outpatient PAG reviews should occur in designated clinics – ideally within the paediatric or adolescent outpatient department rather than within an adult gynaecology clinic.

Designated PAG clinics should be supported by appropriate nursing staff, i.e. specialists or paediatric trained nurses. The waiting rooms and clinical room

for children should have an appropriate array of toys and seating area. The consultation room should provide a sense of privacy and not add to apprehension ahead of the consultation. For example, avoid an examination couch with stirrups and an array of speculums and swabs on display. The room seating set-up should allow a child or young person to feel comfortable being the focus of attention but without feeling a spotlight on them. A triangular configuration between the clinical team, the child or young person and their parent or caregiver is a helpful set-up for the consultation. With the move towards digitised notes care must be taken to demonstrably engage with receptive body language and eye contact. Since the COVID-19 pandemic more consultations are conducted remotely by telephone or video. It is important that the child or young person is present for a remote consultation.

2.3 History

Once confirming the patient's details the team should introduce themselves by name and role to the child or young person and whoever accompanies them.

Ensure you identify who has attended with the child or young person and what relationship they are to them. This knowledge informs and helps direct enquiry when asking the child's or young person's social history.

The team should ask if the child or young person has a preferred name and consider asking for preferred pronouns (e.g. she/her, they/them, he/him).

The PAG team should avoid assumptions and aim to use neutral rather than gendered language. Pick up on cues from the child or young person and ask directly rather than assuming.

With adolescent consultations it's helpful to establish at the start of the consultation that you will ask the parent or caregiver to step outside to allow time for the young person to be seen alone. This allows time for the young person to better explore their increasing

Table 2.1 Psychological development

2–5 years old: centre of their world, objects are alive/enjoys pretend play

6–11 years old: concrete thinking, aware of the feelings of others

12+: seeking autonomy as an individual

autonomy and clinically it allows privacy for further psychosocial history and for the young person to raise concerns they feel more comfortable discussing away from their parent or caregiver. The opportunity for the young person to speak in private to their clinician should also be part of telephone or video consultations.

An adaptive and sensitive consultation model is necessary for PAG reviews with the approach primarily modulated to the child's or young person's age and developmental stage as shown in Table 2.1 [2]. Flexibility is required to navigate who relays the history. As a child develops they are increasingly able to contribute. Direct questions are helpful for younger children, with their parent or caregiver elaborating.

It's important to involve a child or young person in taking their history as this allows for shared decision-making. The child's perspective and the impact of the issue on them may differ from their parent or caregiver. Involving the child or young person will better identify other issues affecting the child including other physical symptoms, emotional or psychological or safeguarding concerns.

Children of one and under are naturally wary of new people and stranger anxiety is a normal stage in child development. Slowly increase your eye contact with them; they will be observing your interaction with their parent or caregiver and will engage with you partly based on their observations of this interaction.

Be mindful that some children will be more shy and prefer for their parent or caregiver to speak for them. Nonetheless it's important to demonstrate you regard their involvement in the consultation as valuable. Occasionally ask them direct questions and allow them some time for reply. Do not be frustrated by a lack of engagement. Reassure the parent or caregiver as necessary that it's OK for the child or young person to be shy.

Particular caution should be taken with consultations where the child's or young person's English is better than their parent's or caregiver's. Have a lower threshold for the use of a translation service to ensure a complete history and that management is explained well to both child or young person and their parent or caregiver.

2.4 Presenting Complaint

Unlike the traditionally taught medical model, PAG consultations are often best started asking general questions about the child or young person to establish a rapport before discussing gynaecological issues – which after all tend to affect their 'privates'. An alternative strategy to this is to ask what the child or young person and parent or caregiver understand is the reason for referral. This will help establish their expectations for the consultation (and indeed worries of what this will entail). This may be an appropriate moment to explain that if examination is indicated what this will involve, with the caveat that you will only examine if they allow this.

When the child or young person or parent or caregiver describes the presenting or referring issue, listen carefully to their words without interruption – clarify points afterwards. In particular check meaning when they use medical terms.

Take time to explore how the problem has affected the child or young person. For example are they missing time off school or hobbies? If so, how much time? How is it affecting their siblings, the rest of the household or family?

Establish a timeline and ask if there were any other changes that affected the child or young person or the household or family around that time. Encourage them to think laterally rather than obvious physical changes.

When a child or young person or their parent or caregiver is talking about an issue concerning genitals it's crucial to clarify terminology. Most children will recognise 'private parts' as referring to their genital area – but this could encompass their entire anogenital area or just be referring to their vulva and or vagina. It's important to use terms the child feels comfortable with – but that the child or young person, parent or caregiver, and clinical team understand these terms to mean the same thing [3]. Table 2.2 gives examples of commonly used terms. Use of a diagram (or a mirror when examining) may be helpful. The child or young person may be concerned that their genitals are not normal; the PAG consultation is an important opportunity to reassure and explain vulval diversity [4].

Table 2.2 Commonly used terms to refer to female genitals

Flower	Bits	Foof	Foo-foo	Fanny	Vag	Cunt
Minge	Nunny	Flange	Pussy	Lips	Woowah	Ninny
Coochie	Shinny	Fairy	Fou	Privates	Front bottom	Tuppence

2.5 Menstrual and Puberty History

The PAG consultation shouldn't be limited to menarche – enquire about the development of secondary sexual characteristics – in particular breast budding. It's often easiest to reference this to school year if the child or young person is unsure of timings.

An irregular menstrual history can be a muddle. Try to clarify the time spent bleeding (shortest and longest) compared to time spent not bleeding (shortest and longest). Many children and young people will have a menstrual diary app on their smartphones – ask if they can show you this if unclear.

Ask about the duration and nature of their bleeds – for instance a partial Müllerian obstruction may present with brown discharge persisting after every period and worsening cyclical pain.

Obtaining an accurate past medical and family history is important both for diagnosis and ongoing management options. Medical comorbidities can be a factor in their menstrual dysfunction or may limit treatment options.

A birth history isn't essential for many PAG presentations but this is generally easily obtained from their parent or caregiver.

Ethnic profiling is inappropriate, but asking about female genital mutilation (FGM) should not be an extraordinary aspect of a gynae consultation. Explain that some communities traditionally practise cutting or circumcision. Ask if they are from such a community and if anyone in their family has been affected? Has the parent or caregiver considered FGM for their child? Or ask the child or young person themselves if they have been cut themselves?

2.6 Systematic Review

A selective approach can be refined with experience. Ask generally about their health – are they their normal self?

Particular focus for a systemic enquiry in a PAG consultation should be on any bladder or bowel dysfunction. This can be a brief question to check no problems – but a greater level of interrogation is required for other presenting complaints or pre-existing conditions such as pelvic or vulval pain.

When were they out of nappies and self-toileting? How often do they go to the toilet? Are they OK using toilet at school (i.e. a toilet away from home)? How do they sit on the toilet (sitting up, legs relaxed on a stool, or leaning forward, reading or on an iPad, with legs together)? Table 2.3 shows typical toileting development milestones.

If they have a complex congenital urogenital anomaly and have had multiple reconstructions from an early age, how do they void? Are they still under urology or surgical follow-up?

Skin conditions can often manifest with vulval or vaginal symptoms and signs. Ask about their washing regime and any personal or family history of skin issues, allergies or atopy.

PAG clinicians are likely to see more young people with eating disorders than other specialties. Ask about their appetite? Is their weight stable? Consider using eating disorder screening questions (see Table 2.4) and where abnormal response take a further history – including diet history, binge or purging, exercise patterns, and their current mental state [5].

2.7 Psychosocial History and Safeguarding

The psychosocial history is important to help tailor management options.

The dynamic between a child or young person with their parent or caregiver and between the clinical team should be considered as part of an overall assessment to consider both any child protection and safeguarding issues as well as the psychosocial component of a condition or problem.

Safeguarding is central to all clinicians and not the exclusive remit of paediatricians. Given the nature of gynaecology referrals the PAG team are well placed to identify child sexual abuse (CSA), child sexual exploitation (CSE), forced or early child marriage and FGM. However, the personal nature of the consultation also facilitates the recognition of other forms of maltreatment, for example physical abuse, neglect or emotional

Table 2.3 Toileting developmental milestones

- By age 1: Most children have stopped opening bowels at night and will show distress if soiled.
- By age 2: Children start to show interest in potty training; a few children remain dry during the day.
- By age 2.5: Children are able to let a parent or caregiver know if they need to use the toilet; they require assistance to manage clothing and wiping.
- By age 3: Children will often toilet on their own; 9 out of 10 children are dry most days.
- By age 4: Most children are reliably dry during the day.
- By age 4.5: Children are able to toilet independently – pulling up and adjusting clothing.
- By age 5: Children will be washing hands after using the toilet.

Note. From 'How to Potty Train', www.nhs.uk/conditions/pregnancy-and-baby/potty-training-tips/.

Table 2.4 Eating disorder screen for primary care

Eating Disorder Screen for Primary Care (ESP)[a]	**SCOFF**[b]
- Are you satisfied with your eating patterns? - Do you ever eat in secret? - Does your weight affect the way you feel about yourself? - Have any members of your family suffered with an eating disorder?	- Do you make yourself **S**ick because you feel uncomfortably full? - Do you worry you have lost **C**ontrol over how much you eat? - Have you recently lost more than **O**ne stone(7.7 kg) in a 3-month period? - Do you believe yourself to be **F**at when others say you are thin? - Would you say that **F**ood dominates your life?
Abnormal responses: *No to first question* *Yes to following questions*	*Abnormal response:* *≥2 yes answers*

[a] From Cotton M-A, Ball C, Robinson P. Four simple questions can help screen for eating disorders. J Gen Intern Med. 2003;18:53–6.

[b] From Morgan JF, Reid F, Lacey JH. The SCOFF questionnaire: assessment of a new screening tool for eating disorders. BMJ. 1999;319:1467–8.

abuse. Be mindful that abuse may be the cause of the PAG issue, or could be happening alongside the clinical condition. Consider protective and vulnerability factors. Ask whether the family has a health visitor or social worker. Discuss any concerns with your local safeguarding lead.

In younger children the NSPCC's underwear rule is a helpful structure to both identify CSA and educate to protect children, as shown in Table 2.5 [6].

Concern about confidentiality may stop a child or young person fully disclosing concerns. Reassure them of confidentiality; that the information will not be shared unless there are serious risks to themselves or others in keeping the information private.

Allow space to explore any safeguarding concerns. Asking about hobbies/what they do for fun outside of school shows that you see them as an individual. This will allow them the opportunity to talk about a topic they

Table 2.5 NSPCC underwear rule

Privates are private.

Always remember your body belongs to you.

No means no.

Talk about secrets that upset you.

Speak up, someone can help you.

enjoy rather than go straight into a potentially difficult conversation on whether they are having sex, if anyone has ever groomed them for sex, or if anyone's ever hurt them.

The HEADSS mnemonic can be used as an aide memoire for psychosocial history. Different areas may be more pertinent than others in different consultations.

An approach to broach drug or sexual history is to ask if any of their friends or anyone at school takes drugs or is in a sexual relationship rather than asking the young person directly straightaway.

Table 2.6 HEADSS

HEADSS	Potential question areas
Home	Who does child or young person live with? Does anyone else live there? Who else is involved in looking after/supervising the child or young person? Any change at home? Recent life events affecting the family/household?
Education	What level at school are they? How is their schoolwork going? What subjects do they most enjoy? Any issues at school with teachers/other children?
Employment	Do they have a job/earn money? What do they do? What hours? How do they get paid? What do they spend their money on?
Eating/exercise	Any change in eating patterns? What exercise/sports do they do/enjoy?
Activities/hobbies	What do they enjoy doing for fun? How do they spend time with friends? Who do they hang out with outside of school? Where do they spend time out of school? Do they participate in religious or spiritual activities? What social media do they use? Have they ever sent any messages/photos that they have later regretted?
Drug use	Alcohol/smoking/recreational/prescription drugs? *Consider using CRAFFT screening questionnaire for adolescent drug and alcohol abuse (see below)*
Sex	Are they sexually active? Have they been sexually active? Do they fancy anyone/attracted to anyone – boys/girls/both/not sure yet? Do they have a boyfriend/girlfriend? Tell me about the people you've gone out with? When did they start sexual activity? What do they mean by sex? What does safe sex mean to them? What contraception are they using? What STI checks have they had? Have they ever been touched or forced into sexual activities they didn't want? How did this make them feel? Are they still in contact with this person? Have they told anyone?
Suicide/Depression/ Mental health	Do they feel more stressed/anxious/worried/sad lately? How are they sleeping? Are they still able to enjoy themselves/have fun? Have they ever thought about hurting themselves? Have they ever thought about/tried to kill themselves? Who can they talk about their worries to?

CRAFFT[a] screening questionnaire for adolescent for drug and alcohol abuse

- Have you ever ridden in a **C**ar driven by someone that was high or drunk (using drugs/alcohol)?
- Do you ever use alcohol or drugs to **R**elax, feel better about yourself?
- Do you ever use drugs or alcohol when you are **A**lone?
- Do you **F**orget things you did while using drugs or alcohol?
- Do your **F**amily or **F**riends ever tell you that you should cut down your drinking or drug usage?
- Have you ever gotten into **T**rouble while using drugs or alcohol?

Two or more Yes answers suggest a high risk of a serious substance-use problem or a substance-use disorder.

[a] Knight JR, Sherritt L, Shrier LA, Harris SK, Chan G. Validity of the CRAFFT substance abuse screening test among adolescent clinic patients. Arch Pediatr Adolesc Med. 2002;156:697–714.

2.8 Examination

In a traditional medical consultation model history and examination go hand in hand. However, examination is not essential for many PAG presentations.

Only examine when you believe management plans will be enhanced by examination findings. Young people presenting with menstrual disturbance may require no examination or only require an abdominal examination. Similarly a child or young person with differences of sex development do not need automatic gynaecological examination. The management of DSD has an ignoble legacy of treating people with the condition as medical educational props, which dehumanises and degrades.

Unless there is acute clinical concern of trauma, bleeding or infection it's not appropriate to perform a genital examination solely in the context of alleged or suspected child sexual abuse (CSA) outside of a dedicated paediatric sexual assault centre. Physical signs of CSA are rare and where present may be subtle. Therefore the clinician examining should be specially trained in forensic examination of children with adequate examination facilities.

The child's or young person's height, weight and blood pressure should be recorded as both an opportunity to help identify general health needs and to indicate an underlying or contributing cause of gynaecological issue. Body mass index (BMI) categories in children and adolescents are determined by age- and sex-specific centiles – where the 85th–94th centile is overweight and those >95th are classified as obese.

Clinical examination starts with inspection, which should include observations made throughout the consultation – including when they were called into the consultation room.

Consider their appearance and outfit. Are there signs of neglect? Are their clothes inappropriately dirty? Remember toddlers are more likely to have food spills and muddied knees as the day goes on. Are they wearing an inappropriate outfit or footwear for the season or today's weather? (Caution should be exercised for those with neurodevelopmental disorders such as autism as this may mean that the child or young person only wears certain clothes.) Alternatively do their clothes or accessories suggest unexpected wealth? Do they have two phones? Could these be signs of grooming or child sexual exploitation?

The core principles of performing physical examination should be observed – maintaining modesty, avoiding discomfort, and hand hygiene.

Only proceed with physical examination with consent and ensure that they understand that this consent can be withdrawn at any point. A child or young person can consent to examination when they have capacity. Those without capacity will need their parent or caregiver to consent for them (see Chapter 15).

Many younger children are curious about their hospital attendance and are keen to be involved; if

there are some nerves surrounding the examination process consider a quick demonstration on a teddy.

The abdominal examination is clinically relevant when presenting with pain or menstrual concerns – particularly where abdominal examination for painful primary amenorrhea could reveal a large pelvic mass representing the hematocolpos or hematometra. An abdominal examination also allows for a better assessment for signs of neglect or malnourishment, and signs of deliberate self-harm such as bruising or scarring in locations that could not be readily explained by falls or accidents.

Safeguarding and clinical indications aside, an abdominal examination grants a physical contact to reinforce the rapport already established rather than jumping straight to genital examination.

All intimate examinations should take place with a chaperone [7]. Ideally the nurse in clinic acting as chaperone will have already met the patient and even if present for the history will not be a new face for the child or young person to meet just prior to examination. A gynaecological examination may have been a worry for the child or young person prior to attending their appointment, and these anxieties are likely heightened by a rushed introduction to a new individual before examination.

Similarly breast examination should only occur with a chaperone. Breast examination is indicated when a child or young person is attending with precocious or delayed puberty, or the most critical observation for signs of breast budding – i.e. Tanner stage 2 or beyond. This represents thelarche and an oestrogen-driven change. Take care not to confuse deposition of fat in the pectoral area in an overweight child or young person as breast development.

Pubic hair (and adrenarche) is an androgen-led change and therefore should not reassure of ovarian function alone. Adrenache tends to occur 6 months from thelarche. Secondary sexual characteristics before the age of 8 should prompt referral to paediatric endocrinology for investigation into precocious puberty.

Hirsutism is poorly defined referring to a 'male' pattern of terminal hair in women. Ethnic variation in body hair is expected, and care should be taken not to mislabel darker vellus hair for terminal hair and hirstutism.

2.9 Genital Examination

The child or young person should be able to remove their bottom half of their clothes in private (e.g.

behind a clinic curtain) – with parent or caregiver assisting younger children. They should have a sheet to cover themselves with before the examination. Adequate lighting is essential for genital examination, which in PAG is predominantly inspection.

Genital examination of younger children is often an opportunistic endeavour – consider examining alongside a nappy change with their parent or caregiver, or on the lap of their parent or caregiver whilst they are distracted by a book or toy. Examining on all fours may be easier for younger children too large for an examination on their parent or caregiver's lap.

In older children and adolescents genital examination can be easily performed with them on the examination couch legs in a 'frog-leg' position (lying supine with feet touching, their hips flexed and abducted). A mirror may be a helpful prop at the examination to help child or young person understand their vulval anatomy and the pubertal changes they may be concerned about.

Pubic hair should be noted and assessed according to Tanner stage.

The entire vulva and perineal and perianal skin should be inspected – this will often require gentle separation of the labia majora and or the labia minora. Your examination should routinely include an assessment of the anatomy and architecture of the child's or young person's vulva noting any skin lesions, excoriations, colour changes or dermatoses. The clitoral hood should not be routinely retracted to fully expose the clitoral glans.

If FGM is suspected the child or young person should be referred for examination by an appropriately trained specialist with colposcopy for adequate lighting, magnification and documentation.

The vulval appearance will differ according to age and pubertal status [8].

2.10 Neonatal Vulval

As a consequence of being exposed to maternal oestrogens in utero, neonates have more prominent rounded labia. The hymen is thickened and can obscure the vagina. White discharge may be seen.

2.11 Prepubertal Labia

As oestrogen levels fall following delivery the oestrogenic effect reduces over weeks with the labia majora flattening and the labia minora thinning. The prepubertal labia minora are small extensions from the clitoral hood and therefore can be mistaken as absent. The oestrogen effects of the hymen are seen over a longer time frame; hymenal tags or remnants may cause much concern – but when later reviewed at a specialist clinic are absent. The clitoris is small (average 3 mm in length and 3 mm in width). The vagina epithelium is thin and appears red and shiny.

2.12 Puberty and the Adult Vulva

With puberty there is an increase in subcutaneous fat deposition with the mons pubis and labia majora becoming fuller.

The labia minora develop and increase in size with more than 50% of adult women having visible labia minora protruding from the labia majora [9]. The labia minora can develop a smooth or serrated edge and can develop bifid anteriorly. Colour changes from pigmentation alteration may occur – particularly at the labial edges. The labia minora can develop asymmetrically especially in early puberty.

The clitoris increases in size (averages 2.5 cm long and 2–4 mm wide). The clitoral hood develops alongside the labia minora. The clitoral hood may or may not fully cover the clitoral glans. The vagina lengthens with the mucosal epithelial lining thickening and becoming pink with rugae.

2.13 Virilised Vulva

With high levels of androgen exposure the labia majora may appear fused or with rugae, and the clitoris may be larger.

Gentle labial traction better exposes the urethral meatus, introitus and distal vagina. Labial traction is performed by both the examiner's thumbs applying gentle downward and lateral pressure on the labia majora.

There is never a need to do an internal vaginal examination in a prepubertal child. If a vaginal examination is required this should be performed as an examination under anaesthetic with vaginoscopy.

Labial traction is also an important aspect of genital examination in young people as it will help identify hymenal variants and help inform where vaginal agenesis or transverse septum are suspected.

Bimanual examination or speculum examination can be considered in young people comfortable with the concept (mainly those who have had vaginal sexual intercourse). Given the advances in ultrasound imaging, internal vaginal examination in those never sexually active should rarely be performed. Similarly, the previously commonplace description of rectal bimanual pelvic examination in child or young person should not be performed unless as part of a consented examination under anaesthetic.

Labial traction allows access to the distal vagina. If discharge is present then this can be sampled with a carefully taken swab – with care taken to avoid the sensitive hymenal tissue.

In sexually active adolescents asymptomatic of STI a self-swab can be taken from the low vagina for nucleic acid amplification tests (NAAT) for gonorrhoea and chlamydia. It's good practice to offer serology screen for HIV, syphilis, hepatitis B (HBV) antigen and HBV core antibody (and hepatitis C antibodies in endemic regions or when the young person is HIV positive).

When a Cusco speculum is used (preferably a small size) then a swab from the posterior fornix should be taken for microscopy, culture and sensitivities (MC&S) for trichomonas vaginalis. A lateral vaginal swab for MC&S should be used to best identify candida and bacterial vaginosis.

When offering an opportunistic sexual health screen you must ensure that you have reliable contact information to allow result giving (and therefore the ability to direct to genito-urinary medicine or sexual health services where positive) and whether they consent for informing their general practitioner if the result returns positive [10].

2.14 Conclusion

To effectively identify and develop management options a child's or young person's participation is crucial.

Each PAG consultation should aim to ensure:

- The child or young person is listened to.
- The child or young person is supported to express their views.
- The child's or young person's views are considered.
- The child or young person is involved in the decision process.
- The child or young person shares power and responsibility for decision-making on management options. [11]

This shared decision model optimises clinical management but also enhances recognition of other psychosocial issues affecting the child or young person. Opportunistic sexual health screens, contraceptive advice, recognition and escalation in cases of suspected CSA or CSE, reassurances about normal pubertal body changes, body positivity, accepting and exploring sexual

and gender diversity are all aspects that the PAG consultation can cover if an adaptive and open consultation model is employed. Remember that all PAG consultations have the power to educate, empower and protect children and young people.

Key Learning Points

- Psychosocial history is important to help build rapport and provide context for management options.
- Ensure consultation time for a young person away from the parent or caregiver.
- Understanding normal diversity is essential for appropriate management.
- Only examine where necessary.
- A shared decision consultation model best identifies issues and empowers the child or young person in their management plan.

References

1. 0–18 years: guidance for all doctors. GMC. www.gmc-uk.org/outcomes-legislation.

2. Levene MI, editor. MRCPCH master course. London: Churchill Livingstone; 2007.

3. Braun V, Kitzinger C. 'Snatch', 'hole', or 'honey-pot'? Semantic categories and the problem of nonspecificity in female genital slang. J Sex Res. 2001;**38**(2):146–58.

4. So what is a vulva anyway? 2018. www.brook.org.uk/data/So_what_is_a_vulva_anyway_final_booklet.pdf.

5. Sieke EH, Rome ES. Eating disorders in children and adolescents: what does the gynecologist need to know? Curr Opin Obstetr Gynecol. 2016;**28**(5):381–92.

6. www.nspcc.org.uk/preventing-abuse/keeping-children-safe/underwear-rule/.

7. General Medical Council. Intimate examinations and chaperones. London: GMC; 2013.

8. Crouch NS. Female genital anatomy. In: Creighton SM, Liao L-M, editors. Female genital cosmetic surgery: solution to what problem? Cambridge: Cambridge University Press; 2019.

9. Lykkebo AW, Drue HC, Lam JUH, Guldberg R. The size of labia minora and perception of genital appearance: a cross-sectional study. J Low Genit Tract Dis. 2017;**21**(3):198–203.

10. Standards for the management of sexually transmitted infections (STIs). BASHH; 2019.

11. Shier H. Pathways to participation: openings, opportunities and obligations. Children Soc. 2001;**15**(2):107–17.

Chapter 3

Normal and Precocious Puberty

Joanne Blair

3.1 Background

Puberty is a critical phase of development during which complex physiological and psychological changes result in the immature child attaining reproductive capacity. The timing of the onset of puberty is related to ethnicity, health, nutrition, environmental and inherited factors. Healthy girls enter puberty between the ages of 8 and 13 years.

In recent years data reporting a younger age at the onset of puberty have been the focus of considerable discussion, and there is still some controversy regarding the age at which the onset of puberty should be considered to be premature. Since the beginning of the twentieth century, a fall in the age at menarche is well documented in European and North American populations. The National Health Examination and National Health and Nutrition Examination from North America reported that the percentage of black girls experiencing menarche before the age of 11 years increased from 4.6% to 12.2% between 1959 and 2008 and for white girls from 2.6% to 6.3%. At the beginning of the century, the most affluent girls experienced menarche at an earlier age than their peers living in poverty, while in more recent years this association has reversed, with white girls living in poverty experiencing an earlier menarche than their affluent peers, although this observation is not reported in other ethnic groups.

While the age at menarche can be accurately documented in prospective studies, data reporting the earlier features of puberty may be less robust. In 1997 a North American study of 17,000 girls reported that 48% of black girls and 15% of white girls had either breast development or pubic hair or both by the age of 8 years. These observations led to a recommendation that the age at which a girl should be investigated for precocious puberty should be lowered from 8 to 7 years for white girls and to 6 years for black girls. However, more recent publications suggest that important pathology may be missed in girls presenting between the ages of six and eight who are not investigated. For now it seems wise to carefully assess all girls aged less than 8 years at the onset of puberty.

3.2 Physical Changes of Puberty

The first outward sign of puberty is usually breast development, described as thelarche. Oestrogens stimulate fat deposition in the breast and stromal and ductal tissue growth. Growth hormone and prolactin also promote ductal growth, while progesterone enables lobular growth and alveolar budding. The distinction of simple adipose tissue from true glandular breast tissue can be difficult in overweight and obese girls, and in these patients assessment of the speed of growth, ultrasound appearances of the uterus and ovaries, and skeletal maturity by 'bone age' X-ray may be required to ascertain a girl's stage of development.

The onset of breast development is accompanied by a rapid acceleration in the speed of growth. Pubic and axillary hair growth (pubarche) usually follows the start of the pubertal growth spurt, although is the first feature of puberty in approximately 15% of normal girls, particularly those of black ethnicity.

Menarche (the first menstrual bleed) occurs approximately 2–2.5 years after the first signs of puberty, and may be preceded by physiological leukorrhoea, a physiological vaginal discharge resulting from oestrogen stimulation of the vaginal mucosa. Menstrual cycles are typically anovulatory for the first year to 18 months, and during this period bleeding may be heavy and irregular.

The Tanner system describes the stages of breast and pubic hair development during normal puberty. This scoring system allows objective assessment of the stage of pubertal development and change over time. Details are given in Table 3.1.

Table 3.1 Tanner stages of breast and pubic hair development

Breast	Pubic hair
Stage 1: No palpable glandular breast tissue	**Stage 1**: No hair
Stage 2: Palpable breast bud beneath the areola	**Stage 2**: Fine, downy hair growth
Stage 3: Breast tissue palpable beyond the areola, breast has a smooth contour with no areolar development	**Stage 3**: Sparse, coarse terminal hair
Stage 4: Areola development with elevation above the contour of the breast	**Stage 4**: Terminal hair that extends across the pubic region
Stage 5: Areolar and breast contour are confluent, areola is hyperpigmented with papillae development and nipple protrusion	**Stage 5**: Terminal hair extends beyond the inguinal crease and onto the thigh

3.2.1 Uterine Development

Ultrasound examination is a valuable tool in the assessment of pubertal development.

The prepubertal uterus is cylindrical in shape and has a volume (uterine length x anteroposterior depth) of 0.8–1.6 mL. The endometrium is not visualised until the age of 7–8 years.

During puberty the uterus descends into the pelvis and increases in size. A uterine length of 4 cm has been recommended as the stage at which the uterus is considered to be pubertal. Uterine artery Doppler ultrasound can also be helpful in confirming the onset of puberty. In the prepubertal girl, the systolic waveform is narrow without positive diastolic flow. With the onset of puberty, the systolic wave broadens and positive diastolic flow is observed.

Oestrogen stimulates growth of the fundus to greater degree than the cervix, and the cylindrical immature uterus attains the mature, adult pear-shaped configuration. The fundus to cervical ratio increases from 1:1 in the prepubertal girl to 2:1 to 3:1, by the completion of puberty. The mature uterus measures 5–8 cm in length and 1.6–3.5 cm in anteroposterior depth.

The endometrium increases in thickness during puberty and menarche is imminent once it reaches 6–8 mm. The endometrium then undergoes cyclical changes once the menstrual cycle is established.

3.2.2 Ovarian Development

Ovaries increase in size during childhood, but remain relatively homogeneous in appearance with few follicles. By late childhood, ovaries have increased in volume from <1 cm^3 in girls aged less than 6 years to measure 1.2–2.3 cm^3 in volume.

With the onset of puberty, the ovaries descend deeper in to the pelvis. Gonadotropins stimulate follicular growth and oestrogen secretion and the ovaries

Table 3.2 Mean ovarian volumes in late childhood and adolescence

Chronological age	Mean volume (cm³)	Standard deviation (cm³)
8 years	1.1	0.5
9 years	2.0	0.8
10 years	2.2	0.7
11 years	2.5	1.3
12 years	3.8	1.4
13 years	4.2	2.3
Postpubertal	9.8	0.6

Note. From Orsini LF, Salardi S, Pilu G, Bovicelli L, Cacciari E. Pelvic organs in premenarcheal girls: real-time ultrasonography. Radiology. 1984;153(1):113–6.

increase in volume and become multi-follicular in appearance. The premenarchal ovary measures 2–4 cm^3 in volume. By late puberty, the presence of large, stimulated follicles may distort the ovary, making measurements of ovarian volume unreliable, but suggested normal ranges are ovarian length 2.5–5 cm, width 1.5–3 cm and depth 0.6–1.5 cm.

Mean ovarian dimensions during late childhood and adolescence are given in Table 3.2.

3.2.3 Pubertal Growth and Changes in Body Composition

The pubertal growth spurt peaks approximately 6 months before menarche. Following menarche, girls gain a further 5–7.5 cm in height, achieving their near adult height 12–18 months after menarche. At its peak, girls grow with a height velocity of approximately 9 cm/yr. Initially bones increase in length, then in width, and finally bone mineral content and bone mineral density. Peak bone mineralisation lags behind peak bone growth by approximately 1 year, and during this period girls may be at increased risk of fracture. Bone mineral content continues to increase into the third decade of life. A number of studies have examined relationships between age of menarche, bone mineral density, fracture risk and risk of osteoporosis in later life. Collectively, these data report that later age at menarche is a risk factor for impaired bone health, but the mechanisms underlying this are yet to be determined.

During puberty, girls acquire fat mass at a rate of approximately 1 kg/yr, and by completion of puberty fat mass accounts for 25% of the body mass. In contrast, accrual of fat-free mass plateaus from approximately 12 years of age. Fat is deposited on the hips and thighs, and as puberty progresses, the waist:hip ratio falls.

Assessment of the speed of growth can be helpful in determining the onset of puberty, particularly in overweight and obese girls in whom the distinction of simple adiposity from true breast tissue may be difficult. A girl's target height can be calculated from the formula

$$\text{Target height} = \frac{\text{Mother's height} + (\text{Father's height} - 13 \text{ cm})}{2},$$

and the 98th confidence interval, described as the 'target height range', rests 8 cm above and below the girl's target height. Overweight and obese girls tend to have a height at the upper limit, or just above the upper limit of the centile predicted from the midparental height range, but grow with a height velocity that is appropriate for their age. Girls in whom puberty is early grow more quickly than their peers during the prepubertal years, and tall stature is then enhanced with the early onset of the pubertal growth spurt, resulting in a height which is above the centile predicted from the target range. In contrast, those girls in whom puberty is delayed are likely to have a height below the lower limit of the target height range.

3.3 Endocrine Changes of Puberty

3.3.1 Adrenarche

Adrenarche is the first endocrine feature of puberty, and describes maturation of the androgen-producing pathways in the adrenal resulting in an increase in the androgen precursors dehydroepiandrosterone (DHEA) and its sulphate (DHEA-S). However, as these hormones have only weak androgenic activity the period of adrenarche is generally clinically silent.

The mechanisms regulating the onset of adrenarche are largely unknown. Adrenocorticotrophic hormone (ACTH) is required as adrenarche does not proceed in patients with ACTH deficiency and those with ACTH resistance.

3.3.2 Gonadarche

The term *gonadarche* refers to the period during which the hypothalamic–pituitary–ovarian pathway is reactivated. Although temporally related to adrenarche, this is a distinct endocrine event.

At birth the hypothalamic–pituitary–ovarian pathway is well developed. Oestrogen levels are high, and gonadotropins are low until the end of the first week of life when gonadotropin secretion escapes inhibition from placental hormones. Secretion of follicle-stimulating hormone (FSH) and luteinising hormone (LH) then increase. Serum FSH peaks at 3–6 months of age, declines from the age of 12 months and is unmeasurable using conventional assays by the age of 2 years. The rise in LH is more modest, and stimulates oestrogen secretion from ovarian follicles for the first 2–4 months of life. During early childhood the activity of this hormone pathway is down-regulated, and it remains quiescent until the onset of puberty.

Gonadarche is initiated when factors inhibiting activity of the hypothalamic–pituitary–ovarian pathway are lifted, and permissive factors enable reactivation of the pathway.

During childhood, gonadotropin-releasing hormone (GnRH) secretion from the hypothalamus is inhibited by gamma amino butyric acid (GABA). A role of makorin ring finger protein 3 (MKRN3) in the suppression of puberty during childhood has been implicated from observations that MKRN3 levels fall in the prepubertal years, and are inversely related to gonadotropin levels once puberty is established. Furthermore, loss of function mutations in the gene encoding the MKRN3 are reported in both familial and idiopathic precocious puberty.

To date, two molecules have been identified that appear to have an important, permissive role in the initiation of puberty. Kisspeptin is secreted from neurones in the arcuate nucleus of the hypothalamus, and the onset of puberty is marked by a rise in kisspeptin secretion. As kisspeptin secretion increases, the amplitude and frequency of GnRH pulses is amplified initially during nighttime hours, and as puberty progresses, during daytime hours also. GnRH stimulates the synthesis and release of LH and FSH from the anterior pituitary. In early puberty, FSH concentrations exceed LH but as puberty progresses and the amplitude of GnRH pulses increases, LH secretion becomes dominant.

Neurokinin B stimulates kisspeptin release, while dynorphin inhibits release. Mutations in the genes that encode kisspeptin, the neurokinin B pre-hormone TAC3, and its receptor TAC3 R are reported in patients with hypogonadotropic hypogonadism and delayed puberty.

Leptin, a hormone secreted by adipocytes, also stimulates kisspeptin secretion. A critical role for leptin in the initiation of puberty has been suggested from observations that leptin-deficient girls do not enter puberty until the administration of recombinant leptin, which restores gonadotropin pulsatility and induces puberty. Leptin concentrations reflect total body fat, and this pathway may have a role in the aetiology of the earlier puberty observed in obese and overweight girls.

LH and FSH work in concert to stimulate the synthesis and secretion of oestrogen from the ovary. In early puberty secretion of LH and FSH is restricted to the sleeping hours, and oestrogen concentrations are highest in the morning, but as puberty progresses this diurnal pattern of hormone secretion is lost.

Inhibin A and inhibin B are produced by the ovary in response to gonadotropin stimulation. Inhibins have an important role in the negative feedback loop, and suppress FSH secretion. In girls with primary ovarian failure, FSH concentrations rise from late childhood.

An increase in inhibin B secretion can be detected before the clinical onset of puberty is evident, which may reflect early ovarian follicular development. In contrast, concentrations of inhibin A, which is thought to be secreted by the corpus luteum, increase later in puberty as an ovulatory menstrual cycle is established.

3.3.3 The Growth Hormone: Insulin-like Growth Factor-I Pathway during Puberty

The growth hormone insulin-like growth factor-I (IGF-I) axis is a classic feedback loop, with growth hormone secretion from the anterior pituitary stimulating the synthesis of IGF-I in a range of peripheral tissues including the liver, which releases IGF-I into the circulation which in turn suppresses growth hormone synthesis and release.

During puberty, the sensitivity of this negative feedback loop is altered. In response to rising oestrogen concentrations, growth hormone is secreted in nocturnal pulses of increased frequency and amplitude, and IGF-I concentrations rise. The mechanisms by which the sensitivity of the negative feedback loop is altered, allowing rising growth hormone concentrations in the face of high IGF-I concentrations, is unknown. During adolescence, IGF-I concentrations reach acromegalic levels, before falling again as growth nears completion approximately 18 months after menarche.

In addition to promoting bone growth, IGF-I also acts on the ovary, working synergistically with gonadotropins to increase sex steroid production, and puberty is typically delayed in girls with growth hormone deficiency.

3.4 Precocious Puberty

Puberty is considered to be precocious in girls aged less than 8 years of age and early in girls aged between 8 and 9 years of age. Girls may present with discordant puberty, with premature pubic hair growth and other features of androgen exposure (premature adrenarche), or isolated vaginal bleeding as the first signs of puberty, or concordant puberty with premature breast development.

Precocious puberty can be further classified according to the state of maturity of the hypothalamic–pituitary pathway. Premature activation of the hypothalamic-pituitary–gonadal pathways is described as 'true', 'central' or 'gonadotropin-dependent' precocious puberty, while puberty resulting from oestrogen or androgen exposure which is not regulated by this pathway is described as 'pseudo', 'peripheral' or 'gonadotropin-independent precocious' puberty. In this chapter the phrases central precocious puberty (CPP) and peripheral precocious puberty (PPP) will be used.

3.4.1 Premature Adrenarche

The term *premature adrenarche* is used to describe a group of girls in whom there is clinical evidence of androgen exposure below the age of 8 years. Adult body odour is often reported first, followed by greasy hair and skin and finally pubic and axillary hair growth. Girls are often tall at presentation and skeletal maturity is modestly advanced.

The presence of clitoromegaly, a clinical sign of exposure to high levels of androgens, makes a diagnosis of premature adrenarche extremely unlikely. Extreme tall stature and more than 2 years' advance in skeletal maturity are also unusual.

American studies report the highest prevalence of exaggerated adrenarche in African American girls, with white Caucasian girls being affected least frequently. An association between low birth weight and premature adrenarche has been reported in some studies, but not others. Obese and overweight girls are affected more commonly than slim girls, possibly due to enhanced conversion of DHEA and DHEAS to the more potent androgen testosterone in peripheral fat tissue. Other proposed endocrine mediators include IGF-I, insulin and leptin. Genetic factors are also likely to be important, and twin studies report a heritability of 58% for adrenal androgen excretion rates.

Premature adrenarche has been traditionally considered to be a benign variant of puberty, but data from a number of different populations suggest that premature adrenarche may be associated with metabolic syndrome and polycystic ovary syndrome in later life. To date the evidence that premature adrenarche is associated with long-term health disadvantage is inconclusive, and further longitudinal studies are required.

Premature adrenarche is a diagnosis of exclusion. The differential diagnosis is given in Table 3.3.

3.4.1.1 Investigation

Measurement of adrenal androgens guides further evaluation. The most common androgen profile of premature adrenarche is isolated increased DHEAS, which rarely exceeds concentrations more than twice the upper limit of the normal range. Less frequently, androstenedione concentrations may also be modestly elevated, but concentrations greater than twice the upper limit of normal should prompt evaluation for congenital adrenal hyperplasia. Isolated increases in testosterone or androstenedione, or increased concentrations of all three androgens occur only rarely.

Further evaluation may require a standard dose short Synacthen test, a 24-hour urinary steroid profile, dexamethasone suppression test and directed diagnostic

Table 3.3 Differential diagnosis of premature adrenarche

Congenital adrenal hyperplasia

Cushing's syndrome

Adrenocortical tumours

Ovarian tumours

Exogenous steroid exposure

imaging, and is most appropriately undertaken in collaboration with a paediatric endocrinologist.

3.4.1.2 Treatment

There is no available or necessary treatment for exaggerated adrenarche, and intense follow-up is seldom required. Insulin sensitivity should be assessed in girls who are obese and those with a family history of metabolic syndrome or type 2 diabetes. Long-term care should focus on weight loss and healthy lifestyle changes where necessary. Girls who are born with a low birth weight may also be at an increased risk of metabolic disease, and also warrant longer-term follow-up.

3.4.2 Isolated Vaginal Bleeding

During the prepubertal years, girls may experience one or more episodes of vaginal bleeding. In the absence of other features of puberty, height appropriate for parental heights and skeletal maturity commensurate with chronological age, the condition is likely to be benign. Basal and stimulated gonadotropins are prepubertal and the uterus is also prepubertal in appearance. A small number of girls may continue to have episodes of vaginal bleeding throughout childhood, while for other girls vaginal bleeding may be a single, isolated event. Most girls go on to have normal puberty at an appropriate age and long-term observational studies report that girls achieve a normal adult height.

However, a small number of girls presenting with isolated vaginal bleeding have a serious pathology and careful evaluation is important. Important differential diagnoses are given in Table 3.4. Examination under anaesthesia may be required to exclude local causes of bleeding including trauma, malignancy and foreign bodies.

Table 3.4 Differential diagnosis of isolated vaginal bleeding

Trauma

Sexual assault

Infection: group A beta-haemolytic streptococci

Vaginal rhabdomyosarcoma

Haemangiomas and papillomas

Exogenous oestrogen exposure

McCune–Albright syndrome

Juvenile granulosa tumour

Vaginal foreign body

Profound hypothyroidism

Urethral prolapse

3.4.3 Premature Thelarche

Girls presenting with isolated breast development below the age of 8 years are described as having 'premature thelarche'. There are two peaks in presentation, the first below the age of 2 years and the second between the age of 6 and 8 years. Spontaneous regression of breast tissue, especially in the youngest girls, is common. Growth continues at a pace appropriate for age. Age at menarche reflects maternal age at menarche, and final adult height is normal. Approximately 10% of girls may progress to true precocious puberty, which may be more common in girls who are obese than those who are slim.

Not all girls with premature thelarche require investigation, but those with progressive puberty, other features of puberty including tall stature, rapid growth, pubic or axillary hair growth, require further assessment. Girls with premature thelarche have a pre-pubertal gonadotropin profile, although it is important to be cognisant of the physiological 'mini-puberty' of infancy and early childhood to avoid over-diagnosis of precocious puberty. Bone age is not significantly advanced, and pelvic ultrasound examination demonstrates age-appropriate appearances.

3.4.4 Central Precocious Puberty

In 80%–90% of girls, CPP is an idiopathic condition. There is often a history of early puberty in mothers. Girls who are younger at presentation, those with rapidly progressing puberty and those with higher hormone concentrations are more likely to have organic disease.

Girls with neurological conditions that interrupt the normal suppression of the hypothalamic–pituitary–ovarian pathway during childhood are at increased risk of precocious puberty. CPP may also result from sex steroid priming of the pituitary, for example in girls with poorly controlled or late presenting congenital adrenal hyperplasia, or following oestrogen exposure from ovarian cysts in McCune–Albright syndrome. Pathological causes of precocious puberty are given in Table 3.5.

3.4.5 Peripheral Precocious Puberty

Peripheral precocious puberty results from sex steroid secretion that is not regulated by the hypothalamic–pituitary–gonadal axis. Gonadotropin secretion is suppressed while oestrogen or androgen concentrations

Table 3.5 Causes of precocious puberty

Central precocious puberty	Peripheral precocious puberty
Idiopathic	Benign ovarian cysts
CNS neoplasia Hypothalamic hamartoma Astrocytoma Pineal tumours Optic pathway and hypothalamic glioma Craniopharyngioma	Oestrogen-secreting tumours of the ovary: granulosa cell tumours, Sertoli/Leydig cell tumours, gonadoblastoma
	Oestrogen-secreting tumours of the adrenal
Other acquired CNS irradiation CNS trauma CNS infection CNS granulomatous disease Primary hypothyroidism	McCune–Albright syndrome Exogenous oestrogen exposure
Congenital Cerebral palsy Hydrocephalus Septo-optic dysplasia Subarachnoid cyst Sturge–Weber syndrome Tuberous sclerosis	
Genetic Gain of function mutations of kisspeptin 1 gene Gain of function mutations of kisspeptin 1 receptor gene (KISSR1) Loss of function mutations of the MKRN3 gene Previous exposure to sex steroids Poorly controlled or undiagnosed congenital adrenal hyperplasia Exogenous sex hormone exposure McCune–Albright syndrome	

are elevated for age. Causes of PPP are given in Table 3.5.

Oestrogen may be secreted by benign functioning follicular ovarian cysts, which appear and generally regress spontaneously. Active intervention is rarely required. Oestrogen-secreting ovarian tumours are rare, and include granulosa cell tumours, Sertoli/Leydig cell tumours, Leydig cell tumours. Gonadoblastomas are more likely to secrete androgens resulting in virilisation. Adrenal tumours may also secrete oestrogen, and rarely both oestrogen and androgens.

Severe and prolonged primary hypothyroidism may present with breast development, galactorrhoea and vaginal bleeding, possibly caused by activation of the FSH receptor by elevated thyrotropin stimulating hormone (TSH) levels. Treatment with thyroxine results in regression of secondary sexual characteristics as TSH returns to the normal range. In contrast to other causes of precocious puberty, patients with hypothyroidism are short and the skeleton may be relatively immature.

McCune–Albright syndrome is a rare condition resulting in a gain of function mutation in the GNAS1 gene which encodes the alpha subunit of the G protein-coupled receptor, resulting in unregulated stimulation of a number of endocrine pathways. The classic triad is of polyostotic fibrous dysplasia, characteristic 'Coast of Maine' café au lait lesions and PPP. Puberty is typically discordant with vaginal bleeding preceding breast development. Sustained oestrogen exposure may accelerate growth and maturation of the skeleton, and prime the pituitary to induce CPP. Clinical signs may evolve over time, and patients may present with precocious puberty in the absence of other clinical features. In this scenario, the enlarged ovaries may be confused for ovarian tumours, and inappropriately removed. Other endocrine pathways may be affected and acromegaly, Cushing's syndrome, hyperprolactinaemia, hypophosphataemic rickets and thyrotoxicosis have also been reported. The heart, liver and gut may be affected, resulting in cholestasis, hepatitis, cardiac arrhythmias and intestinal polyps. The lifetime risk of malignancy is also increased.

3.4.5.1 Investigation

Not all girls with precocious puberty require investigation. Girls who are aged less than 6 years, those with rapidly progressing puberty, tall stature, advanced skeletal maturity and high hormone concentrations are most likely to have pathology, while older girls, those with slowly progressing puberty or a family history of precocious puberty are more likely to have idiopathic precocious puberty.

3.4.5.2 Clinical Assessment

The medical history should pay particular attention to a history of insults to the central nervous system, for example head injury, premature birth, meningitis. New headaches and/or visual changes suggest intracranial neoplasia, while abdominal pain may indicate the presence of an ovarian tumour. Symptoms of hypothyroidism should be considered. Finally, a history of possible exposure to sex hormones in the form of medications or cosmetic products should be considered.

The girl's height should be documented on an appropriate growth chart and compared to her parents' heights as described above. On physical examination, clinical signs of hypothyroidism and syndromes associated with precocious puberty, including McCune–Albright syndrome, neurofibromatosis type 1, Sturge–Weber syndrome and Tuberous sclerosis, should also be sought. The stage of development, assessed using the Tanner stage of breast and pubic hair growth, should also be recorded (Table 3.1). Fundoscopy and assessment of visual fields should be undertaken where possible.

A summary of the investigation of precocious puberty is given in Table 3.6.

3.4.5.3 Imaging

An X-ray of the non-dominant hand can be used to evaluate the stage of skeletal maturity by comparing the appearance of the epiphyseal plates of the small bones of the hand and wrist to reference data from normal girls. Significant advance in skeletal maturity is more likely to be associated with pathology.

Ultrasound examination of the uterus, endometrium and ovaries gives valuable information about gonadotropin stimulation of the ovaries, resulting in ovarian growth and follicular development, and of oestrogen of the uterus and endometrium. Ovarian cysts and tumours may also be visualised on ultrasound. Imaging of the brain should be considered in girls with biochemical evidence of CPP. It may not be required in girls aged more than 6 years with a benign clinical profile. A meta-analysis reported a prevalence of intracranial lesions of 3% in girls aged more than 6 years, but other studies have reported a higher prevalence, and the need for imaging should be determined by the clinical profile.

Table 3.6 Investigation of girls with precocious puberty

Investigation	Purpose
Hand and wrist bone age X-ray	To determine degree of advance of skeletal maturity
Thyroid function tests and prolactin	To exclude primary hypothyroidism and hyperprolactinaemia
Pelvic ultrasound	To assess oestrogen stimulation of uterine and endometrial growth and development To determine gonadotropin stimulation of the ovaries To identify ovarian cysts To identify ovarian tumours
GnRH stimulation test	To determine whether gonadotropins are in the pubertal range (CPP) or suppressed (PPP)
MRI brain with pituitary views in patients with confirmed CPP	To determine whether there is a structural lesion of the hypothalamic–pituitary pathway

3.4.5.4 Biochemical Evaluation

Thyroid function tests should be performed in girls presenting with precocious puberty and short stature. Basal measures of LH can aid identification of girls with CPP, in whom measurements are likely to exceed 0.8 U/L.

The GnRH test measures LH and FSH at baseline, and 30 and 60 minutes following administration of 100 mcg GnRH intravenously. Thresholds at which the test is considered to indicate CPP puberty varies according to assay, and have not been clearly defined. However, LH values above 5 U/L which exceed FSH in a ratio of more than 0.66 are generally considered to be indicative of CPP. Gonadotropin suppression suggests PPP.

3.4.6 Treatment of Central Precocious Puberty

Not all girls with CPP require treatment, as many older girls will experience a slowly progressive puberty which does not result in unduly early menarche or restricted adult height. Key points to be considered in the decision to treat are given in Table 3.7.

Long-term follow-up studies on the outcomes of girls with treated and untreated central precocious puberty generally indicate a good prognosis. Treatment may be considered to maximise adult height, to delay menarche and to address psychological distress. However, the evidence that precocious puberty is a cause of psychological distress in girls, or that distress is alleviated by treatment with a GnRH analogue is poor. The final adult height of girls with precocious puberty is most like to be enhanced by treatment in girls aged less than 6 years. The evidence that GnRH analogue treatment influences final adult height in girls between the ages of 6 and 8 years is inconclusive, while there seems to be no benefit in girls above this age.

Treatment with GnRH analogues has a good safety record, with no evidence of an adverse effect on fertility in later life. There is some evidence that untreated girls might be at higher risk of hyperandrogenaemia in adult life, and to require treatment for infertility. However, it is important to note that data reported from retrospective, observational studies may be subject to selection bias, as it is possible that differences in patient characteristics at the time of presentation that influence the decision to treat may also influence long-term fertility outcomes.

Accrual of bone mineral density slows during GnRH treatment, but there is no evidence that treatment has long-term, adverse effects on bone health and fracture risk. There have been concerns that treated girls gain weight, particularly abdominal fat. However, this observation has not been supported by clinical studies while some studies report a loss of body fat on cessation of treatment.

A number of different GnRH analogues have been licensed for the treatment of precocious puberty, but to date there is no convincing evidence that any one treatment is superior to the others.

3.4.6.1 Timing of Cessation of Treatment

The decision to stop treatment should be made in discussion with girls and their parents. Periods start, on average, 12–18 months following the cessation of treatment, and final adult height may be compromised if treatment is continued beyond a bone age of 13 years.

3.4.6.2 Treatment of Peripheral Precocious Puberty

Treatment of peripheral precocious puberty is directed by the underlying pathology. Girls with

Table 3.7 Treatment of central precocious puberty with GnRH analogues: key facts

Girls above the age of 6 years may not require treatment.

A withdrawal bleed may occur following the first dose of a GnRH analogue.

The evidence that CPP is associated with psychological stress, or that treatment with GnRH analogues alleviates this, is limited.

Final adult height may not be augmented by treatment in girls above the age of 6 years.

Final adult height is unlikely to be augmented by treatment in girls above the age of 8 years.

Fertility is normal in women treated with GnRH analogues in childhood.

Bone health is normal in women treated with GnRH analogues in childhood.

Menarche occurs 12–18 months after cessation of GnRH analogue therapy.

Continued treatment, beyond a bone age of 13 years, may adversely affect final adult height.

McCune–Albright syndrome can be treated with medications that inhibit either oestrogen synthesis or action. This is a rare condition, and clinical trials comparing treatments with these agents and reporting robust outcome data are lacking.

Studies of patients treated with early-generation aromatase inhibitors were disappointing. However, early studies of the newer drug letrozole show more promise with early evidence of a beneficial effect on growth and vaginal bleeding.

Treatment with the oestrogen receptor moderator tamoxifen has been effective for the treatment of vaginal bleeding but long-term effects on growth are less promising. Treatment with fulvescent, an oestrogen receptor antagonist, has also treated vaginal bleeding successfully and slowed the path of skeletal maturation, but long-term effects on adult height are not yet known.

3.5 Conclusion

Puberty is a complex period of development. In this chapter we have considered only the physical changes of puberty. The psychological changes that occur during puberty are equally profound, and the care of the adolescent girl also requires consideration of these complex developmental changes.

Variants of puberty are common and generally benign; however, a small number of girls will have serious underlying pathology and careful evaluation of patients is always required.

Key Learning Points

- The timing of the onset of puberty is determined by genetic and environmental factors and is strongly inherited.
- Although a trend has been described for an earlier age at menarche, the development of secondary sexual characteristics in girls aged less than 8 years is still considered to be premature.
- The normal pattern of development in girls is breast development (thelarche), pubertal growth spurt, pubic and axillary hair growth and menarche. In some girls, pubic hair growth may be the first sign of puberty, and this is particularly true in black girls.
- Premature puberty is generally a benign condition, but in a minority of girls it is the first sign of serious pathology. Discordant puberty is more likely to be secondary to pathology than normally progressing but normal puberty.
- Early puberty may be considered to be 'central', due to premature activation of the hypothalamic–pituitary–gonadal pathway, or 'peripheral', due to autonomous secretion of sex steroids from the ovary, hormone-secreting tumours in other sites or biosynthetic disorders of the adrenal. Very rarely, vaginal tumours present with isolated vaginal bleeding.

References

1. Herman-Giddens ME, Slora EJ, Wasserman RC, Bourdony CJ, Bhapkar MV, Koch GG, et al. Secondary sexual characteristics and menses in young girls seen in office practice: a study from the Pediatric Research in Office Settings network. Pediatrics. 1997;**99**(4):505–12.

2. Sørensen K, Mouritsen A, Aksglaede L, Hagen CP, Mogensen SS, Juul A. Recent secular trends in pubertal timing: implications for evaluation and diagnosis of precocious puberty. Horm Res Paediatr. 2012;77 (3):137–45.

3. Rosenfield RL, Lipton RB, Drum ML. Thelarche, pubarche, and menarche attainment in children with normal and elevated body mass index. Pediatrics. 2009;**123**(1):84–8.

4. Krieger N, Kiang MV, Kosheleva A, Waterman PD, Chen JT, Beckfield J. Age at menarche: 50-year socioeconomic trends among US-born black and white women. Am J Public Health. 2015;105(2):388–97.

5. Kaplowitz PB. Do 6–8 year old girls with central precocious puberty need routine brain imaging? Int J Pediatr Endocrinol. 2016;2016:9.

6. Utriainen P, Laakso S, Liimatta J, Jääskeläinen J, Voutilainen R. Premature adrenarche – a common condition with variable presentation. Horm Res Paediatr. 2015;83(4):221–31.

7. Carel JC, Eugster EA, Rogol A, et al. Consensus statement on the use of gonadotropin-releasing hormone analogs in children. Pediatrics. 2009;123: e752–62.

8. Mogensen SS, Aksglaede L, Mouritsen A, Sørensen K, Main KM, Gideon P, et al. Pathological and incidental findings on brain MRI in a single-center study of 229 consecutive girls with early or precocious puberty. PloS One. 2012;7(1):e29829.

9. Schoelwer MJ, Donahue KL, Didrick P, Eugster EA. One-year follow-up of girls with precocious puberty and their mothers: do psychological assessments change over time or with treatment? Horm Res Paediatr. 2017;88(5):347–53.

10. Kaplowitz PB, Backeljauw PF, Allen DB. Toward more targeted and cost-effective gonadotropin-releasing hormone analog treatment in girls with central precocious puberty. Horm Res Paediatr. 2018;90(1):1–7.

11. Guaraldi F, Beccuti G, Gori D, Ghizzoni L. Long-term outcomes of the treatment of central precocious puberty. Eur J Endocrinol. 2016;174(3):R79–87.

12. Lazar L, Lebenthal Y, Yackobovitch-Gavan M, Shalitin S, de Vries L, Phillip M, et al. Treated and untreated women with idiopathic precocious puberty: BMI evolution, metabolic outcome, and general health between third and fifth decades. J Clin Endocrinol Metab. 2015;100(4):1445–51.

13. Heger S, Müller M, Ranke M, Schwarz HP, Waldhauser F, Partsch CJ, et al. Long-term GnRH agonist treatment for female central precocious puberty does not impair reproductive function. Mol Cell Endocrinol. 2006;25:254–5.

14. Cantas-Orsdemir S, Eugster EA. Update on central precocious puberty: from etiologies to outcomes. Exp Rev Endocrinol Metab. 2019;14(2):123–30.

15. Neyman A, Eugster EA. Treatment of girls and boys with McCune–Albright syndrome with precocious puberty – update 2017. Pediatr Endocrinol Rev. 2017;15(2):136–41.

16. Boyce AM, Casey RK, Ovejero Crespo D, Murdock CM, Estrada A, Guthrie LC, et al. Gynecologic and reproductive outcomes in fibrous dysplasia/McCune–Albright syndrome. Orphanet J Rare Dis. 2019;14(1):90.

Common Prepubertal Problems in Paediatric Gynaecology

Katerina Bambang

4.1 Introduction

There are a number of gynaecological conditions which commonly present in childhood. The commonest of these such as vulvovaginitis are self-limiting though they can be quite difficult to treat. They can often be diagnosed through thorough history taking even before an external physical examination and although most symptoms will have benign causes, it is important to be aware that there are rare conditions which need to be considered particularly if symptoms do not fit into the more frequent presentations.

When assessing a child, it is important to be aware of the differences between a prepubertal vulva as compared to an adult. The labia majora and the mons pubis are devoid of not only hair but also any subcutaneous fat. The labia minora lack pigmentation and have an atrophic appearance. This means that the vaginal vestibule is more exposed to bacteria particularly when girls are squatting. These factors account for a lot of the pathology found in prepubertal girls.

4.2 Vulvovaginitis

This is by far one of the commonest presentations in young prepubertal girls between the ages of 2 and 7. The anatomy of the vulva in a prepubertal girl has fundamental differences which predispose her to developing nonspecific infections and irritation. As discussed above, the labia minora are underdeveloped whilst the labia majora have minimal adipose tissue, resulting in a flattened appearance. This leads to the introitus being open and so with the close proximity of the anus there are minimal physical barriers to infection. This, accompanied by the absence of pubic hair and lack of vaginal oestrogen (resulting in absence of lactobacilli and a more alkaline pH), results in a far less protective atmosphere.

Girls in this age group are often just starting to be responsible for their own perineal hygiene, and so poor practices as well as potentially more frequent exposures to irritants and pathogens in the form of sitting on the ground, playing in sand pits and so on result in higher risk of infection.

The key symptoms in the history may include vulval pruritus, pain, dysuria, vaginal discharge and possibly abnormal odour. It is important to determine the presence of irritants such as use of bath products, scented creams and laundry detergents as well as preexisting skin conditions such as eczema in other parts of the body. Recent respiratory and gastrointestinal infections are also relevant as this is likely to increase transmission of pathogens to the vulva. Frequent episodes of pain especially during the night may signify the presence of threadworms, which are easily treatable.

On physical examination, the commonest findings are erythema of the vulva and perianal region with possible signs of excoriation and occasional discharge. It is possible to take a swab for culture but this is frequently negative. More than 75% of cases of vulvovaginitis are non-infectious, also known as 'nonspecific'. Persistent episodes, particularly if they are associated with profuse discharge or abnormal odour, are potentially more likely to be infective. The commonest causes are respiratory agents such as group A *streptococci, Neisseria meningitidis, Haemophilus influenza* and enteric pathogens such as *Shigella* spp., *Yersinia enterolitica* and *Escherichia coli.* Contrary to popular belief, candidiasis is very uncommon in prepubertal girls so empirical treatment with antifungals should be avoided unless there is proven infection.

It is important to consider sexual abuse in both the history and examination, and if any infection with sexually transmitted organisms is identified then safeguarding pathways need to be activated.

4.2.1 Management

The management of vulvovaginitis revolves around identifying and avoiding irritants and also education about appropriate hygiene as outlined in Table 4.1. It

Table 4.1 Treatment of vulvovaginitis

• General measures	wipe from front to back
	avoid constipation
	avoid tight-fitting clothes
	cotton underwear (don't wear at night)
	non-bio laundry detergent
	avoid washing genitals with soap
	no bubble baths
	wash hair and body standing up at the end of bath time
	dry genitalia thoroughly after bath
	soak in warm water daily for 10–15 minutes
	shower immediately after swimming
	avoid remaining in wet bathing suit
• Medical treatment	soap-free emollients to wash
	paraffin-based barrier creams
	mebendazole if threadworms are suspected
	avoid antifungals unless candidiasis confirmed on culture
	avoid empirical antibiotics unless confirmed infection on swab culture

is not necessary to obtain cultures in the first instance unless there are frequently recurring episodes despite hygiene measures.

These hygiene practices can be time-consuming and improvement is very gradual with relapses if the measures are not maintained. It is important to provide reassurance to parents that symptoms will improve as the girl gets older, both because of development in her own ability to maintain her own hygiene but also because with the onset of puberty will come mucosal changes including a decrease in pH, tissue oestrogenisation and changes in anatomical appearance.

Besides infection, persistently recurrent symptoms may suggest alternative causes such as presence of a foreign body (especially if associated with vaginal discharge or bleeding), which may even just be a small piece of toilet tissue or an anatomical variant such as an ectopic ureter. Any suspicion of the former merits examination under anaesthesia or a renal ultrasound for the latter.

Besides the measures in Table 4.1, it is especially important to spend time reinforcing to parents that

this is a self-limiting condition which in most cases will resolve spontaneously. The British Society for Paediatric and Adolescent Gynaecology (BritSPAG) has excellent patient information leaflets which further support parents with information when at home.

4.3 Labial Adhesions

Labial adhesions are an acquired condition which occurs most commonly in girls aged 3 months to 3 years old. They are not present at birth. They are characterised by variable fusion of the labia minora ranging from complete fusion from the level of the posterior fourchette to the clitoris or partial fusion starting posteriorly and moving upwards. The prevalence has been reported as being between 1.8% and 3.3%, but it is likely a large number of asymptomatic adhesions remain unreported. This is supported by a study where girls had colposcopic examination, which reported an incidence of nearly 39%.

It is thought that they occur because of an inflammatory reaction resulting from a local irritant. In the absence of oestrogen during the healing process, the medial aspects of the labia minora are apposed and fuse partially or completely.

Symptoms reported in the history may be vulvovaginitis, pain on wiping and post-void dribbling or urinary tract infection. It is rare for labial fusion to cause urinary retention and often worried parents will present with a history of an 'absent vagina' noted during nappy change or bathing.

During physical examination, on separating the labia, a thin line is visible where the labia are fused in the midline giving the appearance of a flat perineum concealing the urethral meatus and hymen. In addition, there may be concurrent symptoms of vulvovaginitis in the form of erythema or excoriation.

4.3.1 Management

Up to 80% of labial adhesions will resolve spontaneously within a year of diagnosis and nearly all will disappear with the onset of puberty so management is largely conservative unless there are significant symptoms.

Treatment of adhesions is controversial due to the high risk of recurrence regardless of treatment regimen chosen. As such, management of asymptomatic adhesions is mainly focussed on perineal hygiene, frequent use of emollients and extensive parental reassurance that all internal anatomy is normal. If girls have significant symptoms in the form of either urinary tract infection or post-void dribbling, it is reasonable to consider treatment with topical oestrogen ointment. There is a large variety of treatment regimens reported but the adhesions will generally separate in 4–6 weeks with a reported success rate of between 15% and 100%, depending on the thickness of the fusion. Once they have separated, it is worth continued use of emollients to attempt to maintain the separation although it is reported that up to 34%, if not more, will recur.

Although the oestrogen use is topical, there is some systemic absorption which could result in side effects including breast budding, vulval pigmentation and vaginal bleeding. These side effects are uncommon and regress as soon as therapy is stopped but it is important to make parents aware of them.

An alternative to oestrogen therapy is topical use of steroids such as betamethasone with reportedly similar success rates but topical oestrogen is the preferred first-line course of therapy.

Surgical separation of adhesions under anaesthesia is reserved for severe symptomatic adhesions such as urinary obstruction or in the rare case that they persist following puberty. Unfortunately, recurrence is common even after surgical separation. It is worth noting that it is never appropriate to attempt separation of adhesions in a clinic setting whilst a girl is awake as this would not only be very painful, it would be traumatic for both the girl and her parents.

4.4 Lichen Sclerosus

Lichen sclerosus (LS) is a chronic inflammatory skin condition, which is commonest at the extremes of life. This preponderance of symptoms in prepubertal girls and postmenopausal women suggests a possible hormonal relationship. The prevalence has been reported to be 0.1% in prepubertal girls, and over 15% of these have been found to have a family history of LS in a first-degree relative. The cause of LS is unknown but besides a suspected genetic and hormonal component, it has also been associated with autoimmune conditions such as vitiligo, alopecia areata and rheumatoid arthritis.

LS commonly presents with pruritus, dysuria, vulval soreness and occasional constipation. It can often be asymptomatic for a few months or misdiagnosed for vulvovaginitis, which can lead to progression of the physical signs to scarring.

The lesions associated with LS are characteristic well-demarcated hypopigmented plaques of paper thin atrophic skin, often in a figure-of-eight appearance if there is perianal involvement. In severe cases, it can also present with haemorrhagic bullae, fissures, bruising and petechiae, which can lead to a mistaken diagnosis of sexual abuse, though it is important to remember that the two can coexist. If left untreated, erosion, introital narrowing, fusion and resorption of the labia minora as well as clitoral phimosis can occur.

LS often improves at puberty with 75% of girls noting improvement in their symptoms and 30% noting a change in their skin quality. Some girls will develop a more chronic picture with symptoms persisting and requiring treatment well into adulthood.

The diagnosis can be made based on history and examination and biopsy is not routinely required.

4.4.1 Management

The management of LS is geared at improving the symptoms and preventing long-term sequelae such as scarring and introital narrowing. The commonest first-line treatment is a potent steroid such as clobetasol proprionate 0.05% ointment. There is no standardised regimen though a common treatment schedule is a reducing course over a period of 3 months in the first instance. This should reduce the symptoms as well as improve the appearance of the skin, though the hypopigmentation may remain. Most girls will achieve remission following this but some may require repeated courses. It is important to encourage frequent use of emollients both during a flare up and whilst in remission. If requiring multiple repeated courses, maintenance with a steroid sparing agent such as tacrolimus is used. Side effects of long-term steroid use should be borne in mind and can include skin atrophy, telangiectasia and erythema.

Refractory cases can be treated with the calcineurin inhibitors tacrolimus or pimecrolimus. There is limited evidence for their use but there are case reports of their success. These agents are normally initiated by a dermatologist and do not cause skin atrophy but they do come with a 'black box warning' of a possible increased risk of lymphoma or skin cancer in chronic users so should only be used as second-line agents in those who have failed to demonstrate improvement with high-potency steroids.

LS recurrence has been reported in up to 60% of girls and tends to remit and relapse so patients should undergo regular 6-monthly to annual follow-up to assess progress, and discharge if signs and symptoms have completely resolved. Postmenopausal LS has been associated with an increased risk of squamous cell carcinoma (SCC) of the vulva. It is unclear whether prepubertal LS has the same risk although there have been reports of SCC in young adults who have had LS in childhood. As such parents must be made aware of the potential risk and advised of the importance of long-term surveillance.

4.5 Other Vulval Dermatoses

Systemic dermatologic conditions can have vulval presentations hence the importance of complete examination as guided by a detailed history. Psoriasis and eczema can cause vulval rashes in children. It can sometimes be difficult to make the diagnosis as it is possible for the remaining skin to be spared. Treatment involves steroids and should be in liaison with a dermatologist who has a special interest in vulval dermatoses.

Molluscum contagiosum can commonly present on the vulva but it is unusual for this to be isolated and is most likely to be part of a wider eruption. Bullous pemphigoid causes systemic blistering lesions and is very rare in young girls but when it does occur, it may just present as a vulval rash.

Genital herpes and warts are very uncommon in children. If found in a young girl, there should be a high index of suspicion for sexual abuse and involvement of the local safeguarding team should be prompted immediately.

4.5.1 Prepubertal Vaginal Bleeding

Vaginal bleeding in a young girl always merits investigation and although it is most often not sinister, rare pathology must be considered. There is a wide range of potential pathology so a careful history and examination should help with narrowing down the differential diagnosis. Particular aspects of the history worth focussing on are the duration and nature of bleeding, other associated urinary or vulval symptoms, bleeding from other areas or frequent bruising, history of trauma, any associated pubertal development or a history of sexual abuse.

The cause of bleeding may be systemic such as that arising from exposure to maternal oestrogens, precocious puberty or hypothyroidism but it frequently is localised to the genitalia in cases such as trauma.

Vulvovaginitis can sometimes present with a bloody discharge in a young girl though overt bleeding is uncommon in nonspecific cases. Bleeding is more likely to occur in bacterial infection such as with group A beta-haeomolytic Streptococcus, which will have a raised red infected appearance of the skin. If the history and examination do not point to an obvious cause of the bleeding, then it is worth doing a swab for culture at this point. A positive culture will require treatment with antibiotics for resolution, otherwise conservative measures previously described should be enough.

4.5.2 Urethral Prolapse

Urethral prolapse is the eversion of the urethral mucosa through the urethral meatus, which forms an oedematous friable doughnut shaped mass. It often presents with spotting, which is often mistakenly thought to be vaginal prior to examination. It can be associated with dysuria or pain but mild cases may be otherwise asymptomatic.

Its cause is still poorly understood but there seems to be an association with raised intra-abdominal pressure as it is more common following respiratory tract infections, conditions causing chronic cough and constipation. It is also more common in black girls.

It can be treated conservatively with topical oestrogen and sitz baths as well as managing any of the exacerbating factors above. Resolution can be expected over a period of 4–6 weeks. If conservative measures fail or recurrent episodes occur, it is worth considering referral to paediatric urology for surgical excision.

4.5.3 Foreign body

Persistent episodes of bleeding or bloody discharge with no other symptoms may be the result of a vaginal foreign body. Even soft objects like toilet tissue when present in the vagina for an extended period will cause a malodourous discharge and breakdown of the mucosa. Most foreign bodies in the vagina are small remnants of toilet tissue but other causes have been hair clips, small toys, beads or bottle caps.

Most commonly, especially in a very young girl or if the object is not visible, a vaginoscopy under general anaesthetic is the appropriate management for a full assessment, otherwise occasionally if the object is visible and the child is able to tolerate it, it is possible to gently irrigate the vagina with saline using either a paediatric feeding tube or a small urethral catheter to try to flush it out.

The finding of vaginal foreign bodies, especially if recurrent, has also been associated with sexual abuse.

4.5.4 Genital Trauma

Genital trauma is largely straightforward to identify from history and examination. The challenge is to determine the extent of the injury and also the concordance of the history with the mechanism of injury.

Straddle injuries are one of the commonest types of injuries in prepubertal girls. They tend to occur because of blunt trauma from falls onto furniture or playground equipment. These can be penetrating or non-penetrating injuries. Penetrating injuries tend to occur from falling onto a narrow projection such as a fence post or the side of a bicycle crossbar.

The resulting injuries can range from bruising or haematomas typical of a blunt injury to vulval and urethral lacerations, which may involve the hymen and vagina if resulting from a penetrating injury. If the history is not in accord with the mechanism of the associated injury, there should be a high index of suspicion for sexual abuse and if necessary an appropriate referral made to safeguarding services.

The examination of such injuries should generally be under anaesthetic to assess the extent of injury and proceed with any repair or packing if needed. Superficial injuries can generally be allowed to heal conservatively. In the case of small non-expanding haematomas, conservative advice should include decreased activity, the use of ice packs and simple analgesia. Bleeding lacerations must be repaired under anaesthetic both to achieve haemostasis but also restore normal anatomy. In the case of vaginal lacerations this is sometimes not possible, so a vaginal pack may be enough for haemostasis.

Large haematomas also warrant other considerations such as urinary retention and potential extension into the abdominal cavity so they frequently merit excision. It is prudent to insert a urinary catheter and also a drain in the site of the haematoma.

4.5.5 Malignancy

Malignancy of the genital tract in prepubertal girls is extremely rare but must be considered as a differential diagnosis. The commonest tumour found is rhabdomyosarcoma, which can involve the vagina, bladder or urethra and, less commonly, the cervix and uterus. It appears as a 'grape-bunch-like' mass, hence the name sarcoma *botryoides* (Greek for 'grape bunch'). Children are most commonly diagnosed in the first 2 years of life and 90% of cases will present before the age of 5. If suspected, an urgent referral should be made to tertiary-level oncology services.

4.5.6 Vulval Ulceration

The commonest type of vulval ulcer to be found in young girls is an aphthous ulcer also known as a Lipschultz ulcer. It tends to occur in older prepubertal and postpubertal girls as large and extremely painful ulcers either as single or multiple lesions. They may be preceded by systemic symptoms such as pyrexia, headache and general malaise. Although the cause is unknown, there have been reports of associations with Epstein-Barr virus and cytomegalovirus.

An additional history of oral ulceration should prompt suspicion of a multisystem disease such as Behçet's, especially if symptoms such as arthralgia and uveitis are present.

Crohn's disease can commonly have cutaneous manifestations and these can often present as vulval ulceration. There should be a high index of suspicion particularly in the context of symptoms such as weight loss, gastrointestinal symptoms, abdominal pain and concurrent mouth ulcers. In adolescents, this may be difficult as the vulval ulceration may sometimes precede systemic symptoms.

Treatment of ulcers is supportive with analgesia but may require hospital admission and use of steroids especially if there are any signs of urinary retention. If they are suspected to be part of a systemic condition, then appropriate referral to the relevant specialty (e.g. gastroenterology, rheumatology) is required.

Key Learning Points

- Vulvovaginitis and labial adhesions are largely self-limiting conditions which require conservative management and reassurance for parents.
- Lichen sclerosus is a chronic inflammatory skin condition which can be misdiagnosed for vulvovaginitis.
- All systemic dermatoses, such as eczema, psoriasis and molluscum contagiosum, can present as vulval dermatoses.
- Persistent episodes of vaginal bleeding should prompt consideration of a foreign body or, more rarely, malignancy and merit examination under anaesthetic.
- There is a high index of suspicion for safeguarding concerns if examination does not correlate well with history.

References

1. Hertweck P, Yoost J. Common problems in paediatric and adolescent gynaecology. Exp Rev Obstet Gynecol. 2010;5(3):311–28.

2. Zuckerman A, Romano M. Clinical recommendation: vulvovaginitis. J Pediatr Adolesc Gynecol. 2016;29:673–9.

3. van Eyk N, Allen L, Giesbrecht E, Jamieson MA, Kives S, Morris M, et al. Pediatric vulvovaginal disorders: a diagnostic approach and review of the literature. J Obstet Gynaecol Can. 2009;31:850–62.

4. Mayoglou L, Dulabon L, Martin-Alguacil N, Pfaff D, Schober J. Success of treatment modalities for labial fusion: a retrospective evaluation of topical and surgical treatments. J Pediatr Adolesc Gynecol. 2009;22:247–50.

5. Granada C, Sokkary N, Sangi-Haghpeykar H, Dietrich JE. Labial adhesions and outcomes of office management. J Pediatr Adolesc Gynecol. 2015;28:109–13.

6. Soderstrom HF, Carlsson A, Borjesson A, Elfving M. Vaginal bleeding in prepubertal girls: etiology and clinical management. J Pediatr Adolesc Gynecol. 2016;29(3):280–5.

7. McCaskill A, Inabet CF, Tomlin K, Burgis J. Prepubertal genital bleeding: examinationand differential diagnosis in paediatric female patients. J Emerg Med. 2018;55(4):e97.

Adolescent Menstrual Dysfunction

Meenakshi K. Choudhary and Mugdha Kulkarni

5.1 Introduction

Menstrual disorders such as irregular, heavy or painful periods are common in adolescent girls and may affect quality of life or disrupt sports and social activities and are known to cause school absences in one in four girls. Immaturity of the hypothalamo–pituitary–ovarian (HPO) axis in post-menarchal years is the leading cause for menstrual dysfunction and visits to the emergency department in this age group [1]. Several terminologies have been used to describe menstrual dysfunction, but the International Federation of Gynaecology and Obstetrics (FIGO) system, describing normal and abnormal uterine bleeding (AUB), is the most universally preferred classification [2].

Most menstrual disturbances in adolescence require reassurance and simple measures that can be offered at the primary care level. Referral to a specialist paediatric and adolescent gynaecologist may be required particularly if simple measures fail to control symptoms, in cases of coexisting complex medical conditions or for girls with learning difficulties.

The chapter covers assessment and management of normal and abnormal variations in menstruation in adolescents with key recommendations.

5.2 Normal and Abnormal Variation in Menstruation in Adolescents

The average age of menarche in the United Kingdom has declined from 13.5 in early 1900s to 12.3 years in 1990s [3]. Menarche occurs in the setting of a maturing HPO axis and menstrual cycles tend to be irregular due to anovulation. Cycle length can therefore be variable and erratic although 90% will be within the range of 21–45 days. In the first 2 years post menarche, about 50% of the menstrual cycles are anovulatory; by the third year, these are 21–34 days long in 60%–80%, as is typical of adults. At 5 years, 25% of cycles will continue to be anovulatory, the number decreasing further over the next several years to 20% [4]. Table 5.1 depicts the normal and abnormal variation in patterns of menstruation in adolescents. Understanding of this variation in menstrual patterns is vital to provide adequate explanation and reassurance to the young girls and their guardians and carers.

Delayed or absent ovulation, either physiological or due to polycystic ovary syndrome (PCOS), results in the lack of progesterone and thus its protective effect on the endometrium. The excessive and unopposed oestradiol from ovarian follicles makes

Table 5.1 Normal and abnormal menstrual patterns in adolescents

Parameter	Normal	Abnormal
Cycle length	21–45 days	Frequent: <21 days Infrequent: >45 days
Duration of menses	<8 days	Prolonged: >8 days
Amount of bleeding	Usually 30–40 mL, i.e. ~3–6 soaked tampons or pads each day	Heavy: >80 mL or any excessive loss that interferes with physical, social, emotional and/or material quality of life
Painful periods	Anovulatory cycles likely to be painless Likely painful cramps when cycles become ovulatory, but usually respond to simple analgesia	Persistent pain not responding to simple medical treatment may have an underlying pelvic pathology, such as endometriosis or Müllerian anomaly

the proliferated endometrium prone to unpredictable menstrual bleeding.

5.2.1 Abnormal Uterine Bleeding (AUB)

FIGO recommends the use of the term *abnormal uterine bleeding* to describe any aberration of menstrual volume, regulation, duration and/or frequency in a woman who is not pregnant. HMB is the commonest presentation of AUB in adolescents. A history of excessive bleeding may include prolonged period lasting >7 days, 'flooding' episodes, use of multiple sanitary pads or high-flow absorbent pads, soaking through pads or tampons within 2 hours, soiling of clothes and bedsheets overnight or presence of

anaemia. Table 5.2 depicts the FIGO classification system for AUB based on these four parameters [2].

In adolescent girls, structural problems (P, polyp; A, adenomyosis; L, leiomyoma; M, malignancy) are rare, and the reported incidence of these is 1.3%–1.7% [1]. Anovulatory cycles (AUB-O) are the leading cause of menstrual irregularity and HMB in adolescents. AUB due to anovulation can also be a result of polycystic ovary syndrome, thyroid disorders and hypogonadotrophic hypogonadism such as eating disorders or athletic triad.

Coagulations disorders (AUB-C) appear to contribute to HMB in 5%–36% of adolescents. A possibility of inherited and acquired bleeding disorders should be considered when evaluating an

Table 5.2 Causes of abnormal uterine bleeding (FIGO classification)

Structural abnormalities – uncommon in adolescents	P	Polyp
	A	Adenomyosis
	L	Leiomyoma
	M	Malignancy
Non-structural abnormalities – more common in adolescents	C	**Coagulopathy** Von Willebrand's disease, platelet dysfunction, thrombocytopenia, other clotting factor deficiency, use of anticoagulants
	O	**Ovulatory dysfunction** - Physiological - Thyroid disorders - Polycystic ovary syndrome - Eating disorders - Professional athletes, ballet dancers - Other hypothalamic, pituitary causes–pituitary adenoma, Kallmann's syndrome
	E	**Endometrial** - Endometritis–sexually transmitted infections, pelvic inflammatory disease - Pregnancy related
	I	**Iatrogenic** Breakthrough bleeding with use of hormonal methods of contraception
	N	**Not otherwise classified** - Trauma - Foreign body

adolescent with AUB, especially if the symptoms commenced with onset of menarche. Von Willebrand disease is the most common coagulopathy, with prevalence reported between 5% and 28% among hospitalised adolescents with HMB in different studies. The LoVIC study conducted in Dublin showed that 40% of girls and women with low VWF reported absence from school or work for a couple of days due to HMB; 50% of the study participants had required iron replacement therapy by the time they had a clinical review for HMB; and 70% of women reported their HMB to date back to menarche [5]. A retrospective cohort study conducted by Jacobson et al. showed that despite recommendation by the American College of Obstetrics and Gynaecology, fewer than 20% of adolescent girls who presented with HMB were screened for Von Willebrand disease [6], thus highlighting the need for clinician awareness of the high prevalence of this condition in girls with abnormal menstruation.

Platelet dysfunction and immune thrombocytopaenia purpura (ITP) may also present with AUB post menarche. Platelet dysfunction includes a heterogeneous group of disorders including Glanzmann thrombasthenia and Bernard–Soulier syndrome. History of spontaneous nose bleeds, easy bruising, prolonged bleeding after dental procedures or minor wounds, petechiae and family history of bleeding disorders should be asked for.

Endometritis can also cause irregular heavy bleeding and can be present in association with pelvic inflammatory disease or sexually transmitted infections. Pregnancy and sexually transmitted infections must be considered as a differential diagnosis in adolescents with AUB. It is important to sensitively ask about sexual history. Clinicians should seek an opportunity to speak to the girl in private as often adolescent girls are accompanied by parents or care-takers making it difficult to have an open discussion. All hormonal methods of contraception including oral, implant, depot medroxyprogesterone acetate or the levonorgestrel intrauterine system can be associated with irregular or breakthrough bleeding.

5.2.1.1 Management of Abnormal Uterine Bleeding

Evaluation of menstrual patterns and HMB by keeping a menstrual diary may be helpful for young adolescents. This could be achieved by using simple, free to use, helpful period tracker and period flow apps.

Serious pathology is rare in adolescents with AUB and often investigations are normal. Most cases may be managed with advice and simple medication. Although patients referred to secondary or tertiary care may have tried simple medical treatments, many general practitioners are reluctant to manage menstrual dysfunction in adolescents in the primary sector and there is a need for continuous education and training.

5.2.2 Heavy Menstrual Bleeding in Adolescents

5.2.2.1 History and Evaluation of HMB in Adolescents

HMB is the commonest presentation of AUB in adolescents. Thorough history taking and appropriate investigations (Table 5.3) should be the focus for identifying the underlying cause as has been already outlined.

In a young girl who presents with HMB, haematological investigations should include a full blood count, blood film, coagulation profile including Factor XI as well as screening for Von Willebrand factor deficiency. Specialist haematologist input should be requested if results are abnormal for both a short- and long-term management plan. Other tests such as serum ferritin and thyroid function tests should also be considered.

5.2.2.2 Management of HMB in Adolescents

AUB may present as an acute emergency or may result in chronic bleeding. In acute AUB prompt assessment for signs of hypovolaemia and hemodynamic instability are of utmost importance (flowchart is shown in Figure 5.1). Blood transfusion with or without clotting factor replacements may be necessary if there is haemodynamic instability or if haemoglobin is <70 g/L.

After the initial resuscitation, management should be aimed at identifying the underlying cause and planning an effective long-term treatment. Tranexamic acid is the first line of treatment followed by high-dose oral progestogens. Oral high-dose oestrogen-based hormonal therapy or intravenous conjugated oestrogen is third line but not routinely practised in the United Kingdom

Table 5.3 Investigation in an adolescent with abnormal uterine bleeding

History	Menarche
	Cycle length, duration and amount of bleeding
	Symptoms of anaemia
	Symptoms of easy bruising, nose bleeds
	Period cramps/pelvic pain
	Symptoms of hypothyroidism
	H/o acute weight loss, weight gain
	Acne, hirsutism, scalp hair loss
	Medical/surgical history
	Family h/o bleeding disorders
	Sexual history
	Social history
	Medication including hormonal contraception
Examination	BMI
	Signs of hyperandrogenism
	Pelvic examination in sexually active patients only if indicated
Laboratory	Full blood count
	Serum ferritin
	Coagulation profile
	Von Willebrand factor screen
	Hormone profile: FSH, LH, oestradiol, testosterone, SHBG, prolactin, thyroid function tests if indicated
	Genital swabs if infection suspected: culture and sensitivity as well as NAAT testing for chlamydia and gonorrhoea
Imaging (usually not first-line)	Pelvic ultrasound scan
	MRI may be necessary if Müllerian anomalies are suspected

due to high thrombosis risk. Coagulation disorders like Von Willebrand disease need management with the help of the haematology team. Treatment options include antifibrinolytics, desmopressin, Von Willebrand factor/factor VIII concentrates and recombinant factor VIIa (rFVIIa) in cases of intractable bleeding.

Medical management forms the mainstay of long-term management although most of the evidence relating to medical management of HMB is in adult women and has been extrapolated for use in adolescents.

5.3 Non-pharmacological Management

Non-pharmacological management may not help in the control of bleeding but it is important to advise girls about the importance of regular exercise and healthy diet to maintain a healthy body weight and prevent anaemia. A high body mass index could further cause ovulatory dysfunction and irregular and heavy periods.

5.3.1 Non-hormonal Medical Management of Heavy Menstrual Bleeding

5.3.1.1 Tranexamic Acid

Tranexamic acid is an antifibrinolytic agent which is used in the treatment of excessive bleeding in a variety of situations. It inhibits plasmin and can also improve platelet function. Oral tranexamic acid has an established role in HMB and is effective in reducing menstrual loss by up to 50%. It has been licensed for use in children over 1 month of age [7]. Tranexamic acid can be used both in acute and long-term management of AUB. It is associated with an

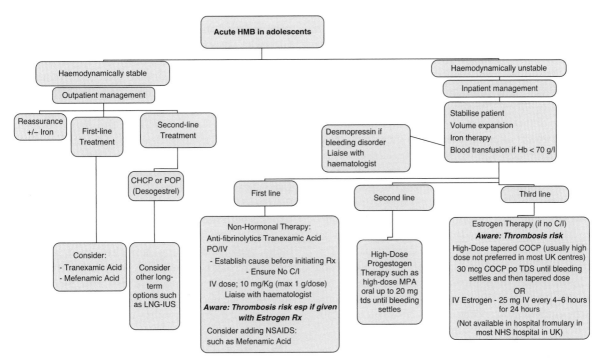

Figure 5.1 Flowchart management of Acute HMB in adolescents.

increased risk of thrombosis and hence should not be used if there is active thromboembolic or severe renal disease, or history of thromboembolic disease in first-degree relatives; and should also be used with caution alongside combined hormonal contraceptives due to the increased risk of thrombosis. Tranexamic acid can be used in adolescents with bleeding disorders.

The recommended oral dose for treatment of HMB is 1 g three times a day for up to 4 days. The maximum dose is 4 g/d. It is recommended to start tranexamic acid on day 1 of the period till reduction in loss is observed or for up to 4 days [7,8]. Tranexamic acid is also available as a syrup or as an intravenous preparation. Both oral and intravenous tranexamic acid can be used in the management of severe acute bleeding.

5.3.1.2 Mefenamic Acid

Mefenamic acid is a non-steroidal anti-inflammatory drug which has been shown to reduce menstrual blood loss by 25%–50% [8]. It is also very effective in the management of dysmenorrhoea. Mefenamic acid can be prescribed along with tranexamic acid or hormonal medication. Other NSAIDs also have a similar efficacy to mefenamic acid for use in HMB. Regular use is recommended from the day before the start of period and throughout menstruation. It can cause gastrointestinal side effects and should be used with caution in patients with renal disease, asthma and bleeding disorders. Most NSAIDs are licensed for use in children over 1 month of age, but mefenamic acid is not recommended by the British National Formulary for children under 12 years [7,8]. However, it is often used off-label to control HMB in young girls at a maximum dose of up to 500 mg 3 times a day.

5.4 Hormonal Management of Abnormal Uterine Bleeding

5.4.1 Oral Progestogens

First-generation progestogens such as medroxyprogesterone acetate (MPA) and norethisterone acetate (NET) are very effective in controlling heavy and irregular menstrual bleeding, and often form the first-line treatment in acute situations. When prescribed as 5 mg three times a day for 21 days (day 5 to day 26), reduction of blood loss by 80% has been observed [8]. NET is associated with androgenic side effects like acne and hirsutism and hence is more suitable for short-term management of HMB. In clinical practice, it is common to commence on NET (5 mg) or MPA (10 mg) twice-daily dosage and increase to three times a day if no symptom relief.

Side effects of oral progestogens include bloating, breast tenderness and mood disturbances. Oral progestogens are also associated with a potential risk of venous thromboembolism, although the risk is more for adults than for adolescents [9] and still remains lower as compared to combined oral contraception.

MPA is recommended as the progestogen of choice over NET in therapeutic dosages as NET is aromatised into ethinylestradiol (EE) after oral administration, thus causing a small increased risk of VTE [9]. Oral NET in dosage as above is considered to be equivalent to approximately 20–30 µg EE. MPA is not associated with aromatisation in this way.

Oral progestogens do not provide effective contraception and they are also not known to be effective in management of painful periods.

5.4.2 The Combined Hormonal Contraception (CHC)

The CHC, which contains a combination of oestrogen and progestogen, is estimated to reduce menstrual blood loss, regulate menstrual cycles and also help to reduce menstrual cramping. There is moderate-quality evidence to suggest that CHC over a 6-month period reduces HMB to up to 77% [10].

Combined oral contraception (COC), commonly referred to as 'combined pill', is safe for use in adolescents post menarche and is an effective first-line management for AUB. The traditional method of use has been to have the pill for 3 weeks followed by a pill-free week, which results in a withdrawal bleed. The COC can now be taken in an extended-use regime or flexible extended-use regime. Extended use or tricycling involves taking active pills continuously for 9 weeks (3 × 21) with a hormone-free interval of 4–7 days. Flexible extended use involves taking the active pills continuously until breakthrough bleeding occurs and then allowing a hormone-free break of up to 4 days before restarting the active pills again. These tailored regimes help reduce frequency and amount of bleeding, and thus prove

particularly beneficial to girls during exams or holidays and also an effective method of contraception. Girls who are sexually active should be advised about the use of barrier methods of contraception for prevention of sexually transmitted infections if they opt for the CHC. Contrary to common belief, CHC is not associated with weight gain or limitation of final height. The risks of CHC are thromboembolism, stroke, cardiovascular disease and breast cancer, and are mainly due to the oestrogenic component. UK Medical Eligibility Criteria for Contraceptive Use (UKMEC) guidance is a good reference guide for prescribers to make safe recommendations for patients with medical conditions.

CHC is contraindicated in patients with thrombophilia, personal or strong family history of thromboembolism, BMI of over 35 kg/m^2, hypertension, vascular disease and migraine with aura. Blood pressure must be checked prior to starting CHC, after 3 months and every 6 months thereafter. CHC must be used with caution in girls who are on enzyme-inducing drugs as this may reduce the efficacy of CHC. Girls taking lamotrigine should be advised about reduction in seizure control. Although lamotrigine is not an enzyme-inducing drug, contraceptive effectiveness could reduce with concurrent use of lamotrigine. It is recommended that such patients have shared care between gynaecologists and neurologists. The overall risk of breast cancer in adolescents is low and CHC will be safe to use. Family history of breast cancer is not a contraindication for use of CHC unless carrier status of BRCA 1 or 2 has been established in the patient.

5.4.3 Progestogen-Only Pill (POP)

The POP is an oral progestogen and can be an alternative to CHC. It has a lower content of progestogen than the conventional oral progestogens discussed above. It is given in a continuous pattern. The most commonly preferred pill is a third-generation POP called desogestrel. POP is not as effective as CHC or oral progestogens in the control of HMB as it can result in breakthrough bleeding but it can lead to amenorrhoea in 20% of users. POP can be offered when there is a contraindication for use of CHCP. Desogestrel containing POP in a dose of 75–150 µg can cause inhibition of ovulation and hence has a longer time window to take the pill compared to NET POP. It is thus more likely to be effective to stop the periods especially as a double-dose pill and is now increasingly used for HMB management in adolescents particularly where the CHC is contraindicated. Desogestrel pill can also be effective in management of dysmenorrhoea especially if continued over 12 weeks. Patients taking enzyme-inducing drugs should be advised additional methods of contraception or to switch to alternative routes of progestogen. Depression and mood changes have been reported as undesirable side effects in POP users although there is no evidence for a causal association. There is no evidence that POP is associated with weight gain and also no particular association between POP and risk of breast cancer.

5.4.4 The Levonorgestrel Intrauterine System (LNG-IUS)

The LNG-IUS is a long-acting reversible contraceptive intrauterine device available in strengths of 52 mg (Mirena, Levosert), 13.5 mg (Jaydess) and 19.5 mg (Kyleena). The Mirena can inhibit ovulation in 25% of users and also prevents endometrial proliferation. The 52 mg LNG-IUS is very effective as a long-term option for reducing menstrual blood loss (74%–97%) and has been shown to be more effective at improving quality of life than other medical treatments for HMB. Both Mirena and Levosert are licensed for the management of HMB. They are also effective in the management of dysmenorrhoea. The 13.5 mg LNG-IUS is easier to insert and associated with less pain but is not licensed for treatment of HMB.

In the adolescent patients, LNG-IUS can be offered where first-line treatments have been ineffective or if CHCP is contraindicated [7]. Patients should be warned about the possibility of irregular bleeding for the 3–6 months and that amenorrhoea is achieved in 65% of users. Girls who are at risk of sexually transmitted infections should be screened prior to insertion of IUS due to potential risk of pelvic infection. The Mirena can be safely used for girls after menarche although insertion and removal under general anaesthetic is required for girls who are not sexually active.

5.4.5 Injectable Progestogens

Depot Medroxyprogesterone acetate (DMPA) and Norethisterone enantate are long-acting reversible contraceptives. DMPA is more commonly used in the United Kingdom and is available as an intramuscular injection as Depo-Provera or as a self-administered subcutaneous injection called Sayana Press, both of which last for 13 weeks. DMPA can induce amenorrhoea in up to 60% of users, although irregular bleeding can occur in up to 50%, leading to discontinuation by the end of the first year. There is an increased risk of osteoporosis with prolonged use of DMPA. It should therefore be used with caution in adolescent girls as 90% of the bone mass is achieved before the age of 18 years. DMPA is licensed for girls over 12 years for contraception if other options are not acceptable [7]. As they are not first-line treatment options for HMB in young adolescents, it is pertinent to review the benefits versus risks every 2 years if prescribed. It is associated with increased weight when used in patients under 18 years with a BMI >30 kg/m^2.

5.4.6 Gonadotrophin Releasing Hormone Analogues (GnRHa)

GnRHa can be used for management of AUB when all other options have been unsuccessful. GnRHa suppresses FSH and LH resulting in a hypogonadal state, which results in amenorrhoea in up to 90% of users. GnRHa can be administered by subcutaneous, intramuscular or intranasal route. A commonly used GnRHa in the United Kingdom is leuprolide acetate, which can be administered subcutaneously at dosage of 3.75 mg monthly or 11.25 mg 3-monthly. Treatment should be offered only for a short time to protect bone mineral density and usually restricted to up to 6 months. However, in certain circumstances if a longer duration than 6 months is indicated then add back hormone replacement therapy should be considered along with serial bone densitometry. Evidence is lacking for use of GnRH antagonists in managing acute HMB and is a future area of research.

5.4.7 Infrequent Periods Secondary to Eating Disorders and Athletic Triad but Excluding PCOS

An eating disorder is a psychological disorder characterised by abnormal or disturbed eating habits; often associated with low self-esteem, anxiety and depression. Three types of eating disorders have been recognised:

1. Anorexia nervosa, in which intake of food is severely restricted

2. Bulimia nervosa, overeating followed by vomiting, catharsis, exercise or fasting in an attempt to negate the effects of eating

3. Eating disorder not otherwise specified (EDNOS) which does not meet criteria for the preceding two disorders.

Significant weight loss associated with eating disorders leads to low energy availability causing hypothalamic amenorrhoea or oligomenorrhoea as the body suppresses its reproductive function to prevent a pregnancy. Low energy availability and menstrual disturbances lead to low bone mineral density and an increased risk of osteoporosis. Reduced bone mineral density is due to increased activity of osteoclasts and deficiency of vitamin D and calcium as a result of alterations in insulin-like growth factor-1, leptin, and peptide YY. Similar findings can also be present in professional athletes or dancers due to heavy exercise and restriction of calories. They constitute the female athlete triad although all three components need not be present.

Management of these patients should involve a multidisciplinary team. Patients with eating disorders should be referred to the mental health team to support with their pathological eating behaviours as well as to help deal with food and body image issues. Female athletes may also need input from an exercise physiologist and a sports dietician. Bone mineral density should be assessed by a densitometry (DEXA) scan and performed annually if low. A Z score less than −2.0 suggests low bone density for chronological age. Girls should be advised a daily supplement of calcium (1000–1500 mg) and vitamin D (1000 IU). CHC can be prescribed to induce periods and treat symptoms of hypogonadism. CHC has not shown to improve bone density in low oestrogenic state. Ethinyl oestradiol in CHC has a dose-dependent stimulatory effect on hepatic SHBG production which may lower bioavailable oestradiol. CHC is also known to downregulate IGF-1, which is a bone-trophic hormone. Transdermal 17β-oestradiol does not undergo hepatic first-pass metabolism or suppress IGF-1 and is therefore more likely to optimise bone mineral density. This can be prescribed along with a cyclical progesterone or an intrauterine system depending on whether contraception is required. Normal physiologic resumption of oestrogen production is essential for the normalisation of the bones [11,12].

5.5 Menstrual Manipulation in Specific Conditions

5.5.1 Management of Menstrual Disorders in Girls with Physical and Learning Disability

Optimal gynaecological management for adolescents with disabilities should be comprehensive; maintain dignity and confidentiality; respect the patient; maximise patient autonomy; avoid harm; and assess and address patient's knowledge of puberty, menstruation, sexuality, safety and consent.

Menstruation in these patients can pose challenges in maintenance of hygiene, coping with AUB, protection from potential risk of abuse and prevention of an unplanned pregnancy. Sexually transmitted infections may be undiagnosed or underdiagnosed and possibility must be considered while taking history and evaluation. Often these girls also have underlying medical conditions including other endocrinological disorders, epilepsy, neurological and cardiac problems, and may necessitate a multidisciplinary team approach.

Effective medical management remains the mainstay of treatment and although induction of amenorrhoea is desirable, it may not always be achievable. The advantages and disadvantages of options available must be discussed with the patient and family considering individual needs. Pills may be difficult to swallow and injectable hormones, implant or a hormonal IUS may need to be considered. Issues like enzyme-inducing medication or anti-epileptic medication or immobility increasing risk of venous thromboembolism should be considered when prescribing CHC.

Although menstrual difficulties are anticipated in this group of patients, premenarchal menstrual suppression is not recommended. These patients may be candidates for long-term GnRHa with serial monitoring of bone mineral density. Endometrial ablation and hysterectomy as last-resort options are generally not recommended without legal and ethical deliberations [13].

5.5.2 Adolescents with Cancer Who Are at Risk of Bleeding

In adolescents, chemotherapy-induced thrombocytopaenia may precipitate or worsen existing AUB, but it should not be assumed that AUB is secondary to thrombocytopaenia.

The potential causes for AUB in adolescents with cancer are as follows:

1. Bleeding secondary to cancer-induced thrombocytopaenia
2. Bleeding secondary to chemotherapy-induced thrombocytopaenia
3. Bleeding related to disseminated intravascular coagulation
4. Bleeding directly related to the genito-urinary cancer

A proper evaluation including examination, haematological and coagulation profile and pelvic imaging should be considered to establish a diagnosis. Acute and long-term management should be considered on similar lines as described above and should involve a multidisciplinary team. A retrospective study described the outcome of oncology patients with regular menstrual cycles who received either DMPA (n = 42), or GnRHa (n = 39) or no treatment (n = 20) before the administration of myelosuppressive chemotherapy. The analysis included only those patients who later developed severe thrombocytopenia (<25,000 platelets/mL). Severe or moderate HMB occurred in none of the women who received GnRHa, in 21% of women who received DMPA, and in 40% of untreated patients [14].

5.5.3 Painful Periods in Adolescents

The worldwide prevalence of dysmenorrhoea ranges between 50% and 90%. Primary or spasmodic dysmenorrhoea (not associated with pelvic pathology) is considered to be more common in adolescents. Anovulatory cycles post menarche tend to be painless unless associated with very significant HMB. Ovulatory cycles are more likely to be painful due to higher levels of prostaglandins leading to excessive uterine contractions which result in hypoxia and ischaemia of the uterus. Dysmenorrhoea can significantly affect quality of life, causing social withdrawal, and accounts for over 90% of school absences. NSAIDs are used as the first-line treatment. There is limited evidence for pain improvement with the use of CHC (Cochrane review 2009). Secondary dysmenorrhoea (associated with underlying pelvic pathology) is seen in approximately 10% of adolescents. Endometriosis is prevalent in about 70% of adolescent girls who have pain refractory to any single medical treatment [7] and noted to be found in 62% of adolescents who undergo a laparoscopy. Persistent severe dysmenorrhoea not responsive to NSAIDs or hormonal cycle suppression warrants investigations. Differential diagnoses for chronic pelvic pain in the adolescent (>6 months) is extensive as listed in Table 5.4 [15].

Assessment of the patient should include a detailed menstrual history, bladder and bowel symptoms, any previous abdominal/pelvic surgery and a sensitive enquiry of sexual history. Pelvic examination may be performed in a sexually active girl and may provide clues to diagnosis. Genito-urinary infection swabs should be taken. Tenderness in the fornices or cervical excitation may indicate infection or pelvic inflammatory disease. Tenderness over the uterosacrals or nodularity may be a sign of endometriosis. If painful periods are associated with persistent pelvic pain consider pelvic ultrasound to rule out other pathology. Magnetic resonance imaging of the pelvis may be necessary in some cases, especially for suspected uterine/vaginal anomalies if an ultrasound scan is unable to establish a clear diagnosis. CHC is effective in the management of secondary dysmenorrhoea related to endometriosis as well as Müllerian anomalies. Other options include POP, DMPA and LNG-IUS. Laparoscopy will be necessary in cases where there is no response to medical management.

Social history should be carefully asked for in cases of long-standing refractory pelvic pain particularly in the absence of any demonstrable pathology.

5.6 Summary

Adolescent menstrual disorders are common and often can be managed in the primary sector with reassurance, simple analgesia and hormonal methods. Management requires careful history and evaluation for underlying conditions, particularly coagulation disorders, which may surface for the first time at menarche. There will be challenges in the management of certain patients who also have complex medical conditions or physical or intellectual disability, and they are best managed by a paediatric and adolescent gynaecologist with the help of a multidisciplinary team.

5.7 Research Recommendations

- A trial looking at the outcome of certain progestogen-based treatments, such as double-dose desogestrel or IUS in management of HMB in adolescents

Table 5.4 Differential diagnosis for pelvic pain in adolescents

Cyclical, associated with bladder and bowel symptoms, dyspareunia if sexually active	Uterus and ovaries	Endometriosis
		Ovarian pathology
		Adhesions
		Infection
Related to bowel movement	Gastrointestinal system	Müllerian anomalies
		Irritable bowel syndrome
		Ulcerative colitis
		Crohn's disease
Dysuria	Genito-urinary system	Interstitial cyctitis
		Recurrent cystourethritis
		Renal anomalies, pelvic kidney
Associated with back pain	Musculoskeletal system	Skeletal abnormalities: scoliosis, kyphosis, spondylosis, spondylolisthesis, myofascial syndrome
Variable pattern	Psychological	Family stress, physical or sexual abuse

- Use of GnRH antagonists for acute HMB suppression in adolescents
- Role of early intervention laparoscopy for ruling out endometriosis in management of adolescent girls with pelvic pain

5.8 Useful Clinical Resources

- Guideline for Management of Heavy Menstrual Bleeding (HMB) in adolescents, published by the British Society for Paediatric and Adolescent Gynaecology, June 2020, www.britspag.org
- Faculty of Sexual and Reproductive Health (FSRH) guidelines on hormonal preparations and UKMEC criteria, www.fsrh.org

Key Learning Points

- Anovulatory cycles due to the immature HPO axis account for most of the adolescent menstrual dysfunction post menarche. By the third year, 60%–80% of adolescents will have cycles between 21 and 34 days.
- Coagulopathy is the second leading cause of menstrual dysfunction in adolescents. Initial assessment must include evaluation for bleeding disorders.
- Sexually transmitted infections and pregnancy should be considered as a differential diagnosis in adolescents presenting with AUB.
- COC is effective and safe for use in adolescents. It is not associated with weight gain and reduction in

the final height as the growth spurt during puberty is prior to menarche.

- Endometriosis is prevalent in approximately 70% of adolescents with painful periods refractory to medical management.

References

1. Smith Y, Quint EH, Hertzberg B. Menorrhagia in adolescents requiring hospitalization. J Pediatr Adolesc Gynecol. 1998;**11**:13–15.

2. Munro MG, Critchley HOD, Fraser IS. FIGO Menstrual Disorders Committee: the two FIGO systems for normal and abnormal uterine bleeding symptoms and classification of causes of abnormal uterine bleeding in the reproductive years: 2018 revisions. Int J Gynaecol Obstet. 2018;**143**(3):393–408.

3. Morris DH, Jones ME, Schoemaker MJ, Ashworth A, Swerdlow A. Secular trends in age at menarche in women in the UK born 1908–93: results from the Breakthrough Generations Study. Paediatr Perinatal Epidemiol. 2011;**25**:394–400.

4. American College of Obstetricians and Gynaecologists. Menstruation in girls and adolescents: using the menstrual cycle as a vital sign. Committee Opinion 651. 2015.

5. Lavin M, Aguila S, Dalton N, Nolan M, Byrne M, Ryan K et al. Significant gynecological bleeding in women with low Von Willebrand factor levels. Blood Adv. 2018;**2**(14):1784–91.

6. Jacobson AE, Vesely SK, Koch T, Campbell J, O'Brien SH. Patterns of Von Willebrand disease screening in girls and adolescents with heavy menstrual bleeding. Obstet Gynecol. 2018;**131**(6):1121–9.

7. Williams C, Creighton S. Menstrual disorders in adolescents: review of current practice. Horm Res Paediatr. 2012;78:135–43.

8. Maybin JA, Critchley HOD. Medical management of heavy menstrual bleeding. Womens Health (Lond). 2016;12(1):27–34.

9. Mansour D. Safer prescribing of therapeutic norethisterone for women at risk of venous thromboembolism. J Family Plann Reprod Health Care. 2012;38:148–9.

10. Lethaby A, Wise MR, Weterings MAJ, Bofil Rodriquez M, Broen J. Combined hormonal contraceptives for heavy menstrual bleeding. Cochrane Database Syst Rev. 2019;11(2): CD000154.

11. Ackerman K, Singhal V, Baskaran C, Slattery M, Campoverde Reyes KJ, Toth A, et al. Oestrogen replacement improves bone mineral density in oligo-amenorrhoeic athletes: a randomised clinical trial. Br J Sports Med. 2019;53(4):229–36.

12. Mehta J, Thompson B, Kling JM. The female athlete triad: it takes a team. Cleve Clin J Med. 2018;85 (4):313–20.

13. American College of Obstetricians and Gynaecologists. Menstrual manipulation for adolescents with physical and developmental disabilities. Committee Opinion 668. 2016.

14. Meirow D, Rabinovici J, Katz D, Or R, Shufaro Y, Ben-Yehuda D. Prevention of severe menorrhagia in oncology patients with treatment-induced thrombocytopenia by luteinizing hormone-releasing hormone agonist and depo-medroxyprogesterone acetate. Cancer. 2006;107:1634.

15. Hickey M, Balen A. Menstrual disorders in adolescence: investigation and management. Hum Reprod Update. 2003;9(5):493–504.

Polycystic Ovary Syndrome in Adolescence

Adam H. Balen

6.1 Introduction

The polycystic ovary syndrome (PCOS) is a common condition, affecting 10%–15% of women, and is defined by the presence of at least two of the following three criteria (Table 6.1): (1) a menstrual cycle disturbance, that is oligomenorrhoea or amenorrhoea, (2) evidence of hyperandrogenism, as assessed by either physical signs (excess hair growth on the face or body (hirsutism), acne, alopecia) or a biochemical elevation of androgens, and/or (3) polycystic ovaries as seen by ultrasound scan, after appropriate endocrine tests have been carried out to rule out other causes of androgen excess and menstrual cycle irregularity. PCOS therefore encompasses many of the natural features experienced by adolescent girls and so it is important to ensure that an appropriate diagnosis is made. Indeed, for this reason, the current guidelines suggest that the diagnosis of PCOS cannot be made until at least 3 years after menarche and some even suggest that one should wait for 8 years, which is when full reproductive maturity has usually been attained. It is important that adolescents are properly educated about the natural changes during puberty so that they have a full understanding of how their bodies work and their reproductive health and what to do if things are not right.

Table 6.1 Diagnosis of PCOS

Two of the following are required:
1. Menstrual cycle disturbance, that is, oligomenorrhoea or amenorrhoea
2. Hyperandrogenism: either physical signs of hirsutism, acne or alopecia or a biochemical elevation of androgens (usually testosterone)
3. Polycystic ovaries on ultrasound scan
After a full endocrine profile to rule out other causes of androgen excess and menstrual cycle irregularity.

6.2 Diagnosis of PCOS in Adolescence

The polycystic ovary syndrome (PCOS) is a condition with a heterogeneous collection of signs and symptoms that gathered together form a spectrum of a disorder with a mild presentation in some, whilst in others there may be a severe disturbance of reproductive, endocrine and metabolic function. The aetiology and pathophysiology of PCOS is multifactorial, with genetic and environmental factors that influence in utero development of the hypothalamic–pituitary–ovarian axis, ovarian function, fat deposition and adipocyte function, and insulin metabolism. Furthermore, there are ethnic variations in presentation, with some ethnicities exhibiting a greater degree of hirsutism (e.g. South Asians compared with East Asians).

For most the syndrome usually evolves during adolescence, there is considerable heterogeneity of symptoms in those with PCOS and for an individual these may change over time. Polycystic ovaries can even exist without clinical signs of the syndrome, and this is a common finding during adolescence when the ovaries naturally have a high number of follicles. Using modern, high-resolution ultrasound technology, the consensus for the morphology of the polycystic ovary has been defined as an ovary with 20 or more follicles measuring 2–9 mm in diameter and/or increased ovarian volume (>10 cm^3), although this assessment can only realistically be made in adult women and age-specific cut-offs for the definition of the polycystic ovary have not yet been agreed for adolescent girls. Furthermore, an abdominal ultrasound scan rather than a trans-vaginal scan is usually required in adolescent girls, when an ovarian volume of greater than 10 cm^3 is considered likely to represent the present of polycystic ovaries.

Menstrual disturbance, usually oligomenorrhea and sometimes primary or secondary amenorrhea, is one of the key features of PCOS in the adult (Table 6.2). However, in adolescence, menstrual irregularities are

Table 6.2 Definition of an irregular menstrual cycle

- Normal in the first year post menarche as part of the pubertal transition
- 1 to <3 years post menarche: <21 or >45 days
- 3 years post menarche to perimenopause: <21 or >35 days or <8 cycles per year
- 1 year post menarche: >90 days for any one cycle
- Primary amenorrhea by age 15 or >3 years post-thelarche (breast development)

very common with between 40–85% having anovulatory cycles. There is a progression towards more ovulatory cycles with increasing gynaecological age (that is age after menarche), increasing from 23%–35% during the first year after menarche to 63%–65% by 5 years after menarche. It has been suggested that half of adolescent girls who have persistent oligomenorrhea or secondary amenorrhea beyond 2 years after menarche are affected by a permanent ovulatory disorder. Various factors influence ovarian function, in particular an individual's body weight and nutritional status.

Acne is common during the adolescent years and in most subjects is a transitory phenomenon that correlates poorly with circulating hormone levels. Hirsutism may be a better marker of hyperandrogenism, and progressive hirsutism during the adolescent years may be an important sign of PCOS. Biochemical markers, predominantly an elevated serum testosterone concentration, may also vary and do not correlate well with clinical signs.

There are a number of interlinking factors that may affect expression of PCOS. For example, a gain in weight is associated with a worsening of symptoms whilst weight loss may ameliorate the endocrine and metabolic profile and symptomatology. The features of obesity, hyperinsulinaemia and hyperandrogenaemia which are commonly seen in PCOS are also known to be factors which confer an increased risk of cardiovascular disease and non-insulin-dependent diabetes mellitus (type 2 DM).

There is no agreement concerning how to diagnose PCOS in adolescence. In fact, during the transition of girls into adulthood, several features may be in evolution or may only be transitory findings. If there are features suggestive of PCOS then a tentative diagnosis may be assumed and discussed with the patient and her parents. Management should be orientated towards the symptoms she is experiencing and lifestyle advice given (see below). When the diagnosis cannot be confirmed, the individual should be followed closely until adulthood, and the diagnosis should be re-considered if the symptoms persist.

6.2.1 Examination

Measurement of height and weight should be performed in order to calculate the patient's body mass index (BMI). The normal range is 20–25 kg/m^2, although this is only applicable once adult height has been attained and so may not be appropriate during early adolescence, when paediatric growth charts should be used.

Signs of hyperandrogenism – acne, hirsutism, alopecia – are suggestive of PCOS, and biochemical screening helps to differentiate other causes of androgen excess. It is important to distinguish between hyperandrogenism and virilisation, which also occurs with higher circulating androgen levels than seen in PCOS and leads to deepening of the voice, breast atrophy, increase in muscle bulk and cliteromegaly. A rapid onset of hirsutism suggests the possibility of an androgen-secreting tumour of the ovary or adrenal gland, although these are very rare.

Hirsutism is characterised by terminal hair growth in a male pattern of distribution (Figure 6.1), including the chin, upper lip, chest, upper and lower back, upper and lower abdomen, upper arm, thigh and buttocks. A standardised scoring system, such as the modified Ferriman–Gallwey score (Figure 6.2), may be used, with a level ≥4–6 indicating hirsutism. Such a pictorial score is useful for monitoring the progress of hirsutism, or its response to treatment. It should be remembered, however, that not all hair on the body is necessarily responsive to hormone changes (e.g. the upper thighs). There may also be big ethnic variations in the expression of hirsutism, with women from South Asia and Mediterranean countries often having more pronounced presentation. whereas those from the Far East may not have much in the way of bodily hair. Furthermore, the degree of hirsutism does not correlate that well with the actual levels of circulating androgens.

Alopecia is uncommon during adolescence and is a very distressing symptom. It may be associated with iron deficiency and other nutritional deficiencies and so malabsorptive syndromes such as coeliac disease should also be excluded.

Acne is common in adolescents and a pictorial score may also be kept, although there isn't a universally agreed classification. Acanthosis nigricans is a sign of profound insulin resistance and is usually visible as hyperpigmented thickening of the skin folds of the axilla and neck and is associated with PCOS and obesity

6.2.2 Investigations

A measurement of total testosterone is considered adequate for general screening. It is unnecessary to measure other androgens unless total testosterone is above the 95th percentile of your local assay. Insulin resistance occurs in those who are overweight and insulin suppresses the production of sex hormone–binding globulin (SHBG) by the liver, resulting in a high free androgen index (calculated by (testosterone / SHBG) x 100) in the presence of a normal total testosterone. The measurement of SHBG is not required in routine practice but is a useful surrogate marker for insulin resistance.

Late-onset congenital adrenal hyperplasia (CAH) presents with features very similar to those of PCOS and so in populations where CAH is more prevalent a measurement of 17-hydroxy-progesterone should be performed. One should also be aware of the possibility of Cushing's syndrome in those with features of PCOS and obesity as it is a disease of insidious onset and dire consequences, although uncommon in adolescents; additional clues are the presence of central obesity, moon face, plethoric complexion, buffalo hump,

---

Only terminal hairs should be considered in pathological hirsutism.

Terminal hairs >5 mm in length vary in shape and texture and are usually pigmented.

Over-estimation of hirsutism may occur if vellus hair is confused with terminal hair–ethnic variation in vellus hair density.

Figure 6.1 Hirsutism.

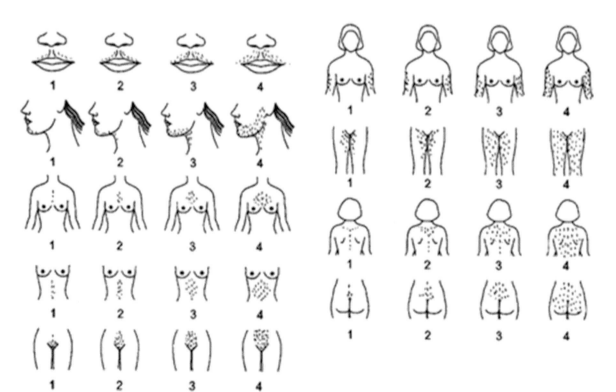

Figure 6.2 Ferriman–Gallwey score.

Table 6.3 Gonadatrophin levels in amenorrhoea or oligomenorrhoea

Diagnosis of other causes of menstrual irregularity

	FSH	LH	Oestradiol
PCOS	normal	↑ or normal	normal
Ovarian insufficiency / menopause:	↑	↑	↓
Hypothalamic or pituitary problems: underweight, over-exercise, chronic illness	↓	↓	↓

also measure TFTs, Prolactin

proximal myopathy, thin skin, bruising and abdominal striae (which alone are a common finding in obese individuals).

Serum gonadotrophin measurements help to distinguish between causes of menstrual irregularity (Table 6.3). PCOS is associated with normal levels of follicle-stimulating hormone (FSH) and luteinising hormone (LH) levels that are either normal or elevated. Those with hypothalamic amenorrhoea have low levels of FSH and LH whilst they will be elevated in those with premature ovarian insufficiency. Serum measurements of oestradiol may vary considerably, although they tend to be low in all causes of amenorrhoea other than PCOS. If the patient is well oestrogenised, the endometrium will be clearly seen on an ultrasound scan and should be shed in response to a short course of a progestogen (e.g. medroxyprogesterone acetate 20 mg daily for 7 days).

Anti-Müllerian hormone (AMH) is best known as a product of the testes during fetal development that suppresses the development of Müllerian structures. AMH is also produced by the pre-antral and antral follicles and is a good marker of ovarian reserve. The presence of polycystic ovaries is associated with high serum AMH concentrations.

Adolescent girls with PCOS may have insulin resistance and impaired glucose tolerance, especially if they are overweight. Whilst associated with elevated serum concentrations of insulin this is not measured in clinical practice, instead either an oral glucose

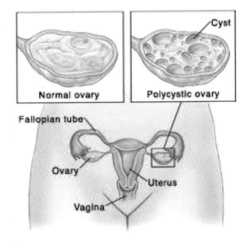

Figure 6.3 Gonadatrophin levels in amenorrhoea or oligomenorrhoea.

tolerance test may be performed to screen for diabetes and impaired glucose tolerance or, more commonly, a measurement of HbA1 c is taken.

Polycystic ovaries are commonly detected by ultrasound (Figure 6.3), with estimates of the prevalence in the general population being in the order of 20%–33%. The eponymous 'cysts' are in reality immature egg-containing follicles whose development has been arrested. The actual number of cysts to define the polycystic ovary should be at least 20 per ovary in adult women (Figure 6.4) but, as already stated, this number is likely to be much higher during adolescent years and age-related cut-off values have not been agreed, making it difficult to confirm the diagnosis during adolescence. Furthermore, a transabdominal scan (Figure 6.5) rather than a trans-vaginal scan (Figure 6.4) is more appropriate in adolescence, when an ovarian volume of greater than 10 cm^3 suggests the presence of polycystic ovaries.

6.3 Management of Polycystic Ovary Syndrome

6.3.1 Psychological Well-being and Quality of Life

The clinical management of a young woman with PCOS should be focussed on her individual problems. It is important to appreciate that all aspects of the syndrome may have a significant impact on psychological well-

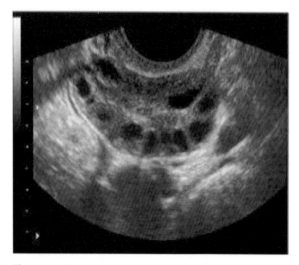

Figure 6.4 Trans-vaginal ultrasound scan of a polycystic ovary.

being and quality of life, in particular the dermatological manifestations and obesity. Furthermore, there is an increased prevalence of eating disorders and disordered eating patterns associated with PCOS, in particular anorexia nervosa and bulimia.

If eating disorders and disordered eating are suspected, further assessment, referral and treatment, including psychological therapy, should be offered by appropriately trained health professionals. Psychological factors such as anxiety, depressive symptoms and body image concerns require careful management and support to optimise engagement and adherence to lifestyle interventions.

6.3.2 Obesity

Being overweight worsens both symptomatology and the endocrine profile. Clinical features are likely to improve with weight loss, although this can be hard to achieve and requires significant support both from the clinical team and family. Lifestyle factors are often of familial origin and so it may be helpful to coach the whole family and in particular the patient's parents. Healthy lifestyle behaviours encompassing healthy eating and regular physical activity should be recommended to achieve and/or maintain healthy weight and to optimise hormonal outcomes, general health and quality of life.

The right diet for an individual is one that is practical, sustainable and compatible with her lifestyle. It is sensible to keep carbohydrate content down and to avoid excess fatty foods. It is often helpful to refer to a dietician. Bariatric surgery (either gastric banding or gastric bypass) is sometimes required, although rarely performed during adolescence.

6.3.3 Menstrual Irregularity

Amenorrhoeic adolescents with PCOS are not oestrogen deficient and are not at risk of osteoporosis. Indeed, they

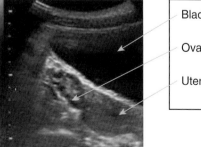

Bladder

Ovary

Uterus

Figure 6.5 Transabdominal ultrasound scan of a polycystic ovary.

have unopposed oestrogen as they are not ovulating and so are at risk of endometrial hyperplasia, which may progress to endometrial adenocarcinoma over time. It is inadvisable for an individual with PCOS to go more than 90 days without a bleed and so some form of endometrial protection is required. The easiest way to control the menstrual cycle is the use of a low-dose combined oral contraceptive preparation. This will result in an artificial cycle and regular shedding of the endometrium. An alternative is a progestogen such as medroxyprogesterone acetate (Provera) for 12 days every 1–3 months to induce a withdrawal bleed, or the continuous provision of progesterone into the uterine cavity by a Mirena, or equivalent, intrauterine system.

6.3.4 Hyperandrogenism and Hirsutism

The treatment of hirsutism and acne will depend very much upon the degree to which the adolescent sees this as a concern. There is significant psychological morbidity associated with these problems and so support is essential in order to manage expectations. Drug therapies may take 6–9 months or longer before any improvement in hirsutism is perceived. During this time physical treatments including electrolysis, waxing and bleaching may be helpful. Electrolysis is time consuming, painful and expensive and should be performed by an expert practitioner. Regrowth is not uncommon and there is no really permanent cosmetic treatment. Laser and photothermolysis techniques are more expensive but may have a longer duration of effect. Repeated treatments are required because only hair follicles in the growing phase are obliterated at each treatment. Hair growth occurs in three cycles, so 6–9 months of regular treatments are necessary. The topical use of eflornithine may be effective as it inhibits the enzyme ornithine decarboxylase in hair follicles and may be a useful therapy for those who wish to avoid hormonal treatments, but may also be used in conjunction with hormonal therapy. Eflornithine may cause some thinning of the skin and so high-factor sun block is recommended when exposed to the sun.

The COCP may be prescribed both for the management of hyperandrogenism and irregular menstrual cycles and is also appropriate for adolescents who are considered to be 'at risk' but not yet diagnosed with PCOS. The various COCP preparations have similar efficacy in treating hirsutism and so the lowest effective oestrogen doses (such as 20–30 µg of ethinyloestradiol or equivalent) should be prescribed. The effect on acne and seborrhoea is usually evident within a couple of months of commencing a COCP whilst hirsutism may take 6–9 months to improve.

While almost all of the COCPs contain ethinyloestradiol the progestogens vary in their androgenic potential. Norethindrone, norgestrel and levonorgestrel are known to have androgenic activity, whereas desogestrel, norgestimate and gestodene are less androgenic and so are preferable in the management of PCOS. COCPs containing progestins with anti-androgenic activity (cyproterone acetate, drospirenone) have not been shown to have superior efficacy. And so, whilst traditionally the 35 µg ethinyloestradiol plus cyproterone acetate preparations have been used in the management of PCOS, there is no evidence of superior efficacy and so they should not be considered first line in PCOS, due to adverse effects including venous thromboembolic risks.

The contraindications and side effects of COCPs need to be considered in particular for those with PCOS-specific risk factors such as high BMI, hyperlipidemia and hypertension. In those for whom the combined oral contraceptive pill is contraindicated, spironolactone, a weak diuretic with anti-androgenic properties, may be used at a daily dose of 25–100 mg in those over 16 and monitored carefully. Contraception should be advised if required as spironolactone may have an adverse effect on the developing fetus. Other anti-androgens (e.g. ketoconazole, finasteride and flutamide) are not appropriate in adolescents due to their adverse side effects.

Metformin, may also be of benefit in adolescence because of the coexistence of the hyperinsulinaemia related to puberty and PCOS, particularly in those identified with impaired glucose tolerance.

6.3.5 Infertility

Fertility is not usually a concern of the adolescent girl with PCOS, but the question is often asked by concerned parents. Essentially maintaining a healthy lifestyle and a normal body weight will lessen the likelihood of problems when fertility is required. Ovulation induction therapies may be needed in the future including letrozole, clomiphene citrate gonadotrophin therapy or laparoscopic ovarian diathermy. Women with PCOS are at risk of ovarian hyperstimulation syndrome (OHSS) and multiple pregnancy, and so ovulation induction has to be carefully monitored with serial ultrasound scans. Improvements in lifestyle, with a combination of exercise and diet to achieve weight reduction, are important for improving the prospects of both natural and drug-induced ovulation. In addition, overweight women with PCOS are at increased risk of miscarriage and obstetric complications, such as gestational diabetes and pre-eclampsia.

6.4 Long-Term Health Consequences of Polycystic Ovary Syndrome

There have been a large number of studies demonstrating the presence of insulin resistance and corresponding hyperinsulinaemia in both obese and non-obese women and girls with PCOS. This leads to an increased risk for type 2 diabetes and also potentially for cardiovascular disease. Women with PCOS who are oligomenorrhoeic are more likely to be insulin resistant than those with regular cycles, irrespective of their BMI, with the inter-menstrual interval correlating with the degree of insulin resistance.

Women with PCOS have a greater truncal abdominal fat distribution as demonstrated by a higher waist to hip ratio ('central obesity'). The central distribution of fat is independent of BMI and associated with higher plasma insulin and triglyceride concentrations and reduced high-density lipoprotein (HDL) cholesterol concentrations. From a practical point of view, if the measurement of waist circumference is greater than 80 cm, there will be excess visceral fat and an increased risk of metabolic problems.

All those with PCOS should be offered regular monitoring for weight changes and excess weight, at a minimum of 6–12 monthly. Overweight and obese women with PCOS, regardless of age, should have a fasting lipid profile (cholesterol, low-density lipoprotein cholesterol, high-density lipoprotein cholesterol and triglyceride level at diagnosis). Thereafter, frequency of measurement should be based on the presence of hyperlipidemia and cardiovascular risk factors (family history, obesity, cigarette smoking, dyslipidemia, hypertension, impaired glucose tolerance and lack of physical activity).

Consideration should also be taken for an increased risk of endometrial adenocarcinoma in those with a history of chronic amenorrhoea and obesity.

Key Learning Points

- PCOS is difficult to diagnose in adolescence, as many of the symptoms occur naturally, and so a firm diagnosis may not be possible until up to 8 years after menarche.

- PCOS is a heterogeneous condition. Diagnosis is made by the presence of two of the following three criteria: (1) oligo-ovulation and/or anovulation, (2) hyperandrogenism (clinical and/or biochemical) or (3) polycystic ovaries, with the exclusion of other aetiologies of menstrual irregularity and androgen excess.

- Management is symptom orientated, and a pragmatic approach is required during adolescent years.

- If obese, weight loss improves symptoms and endocrinology and should be encouraged. Dietary advice and exercise are essential components of a weight-reduction programme.

- A programme of long-term health surveillance is advisable.

References

1. Balen AH. Polycystic ovary syndrome. Obstetr Gynaecol. 2017;**19**(2):119–29.

2. Teede HJ, Misso ML, Costello MF, Dokras A, Laven J, Misso ML, et al. Recommendations from the international evidence-based guideline for the assessment and management of polycystic ovary syndrome. Fertil Steri. 2018;**110**:364–79; Clin Endocrinol. 2018;**89**:251–68; Hum Reprod. 2018;**33**:1602–18. Simultaneous publications.

3. Fauser B, Tarlatzis B, Chang J, Azziz R, Legro R, Dewailly D, et al. Revised 2003 consensus on diagnostic criteria and long-term health risks related to polycystic ovary syndrome (PCOS). Hum Reprod. 2004;**19**:41–7.

4. Fauser BCJM, Tarlatzis BC, Rerbar RW, Legro RS, Balen AH, Lobo R, et al. Consensus on women's health aspects of polycystic ovary syndrome (PCOS): the Amsterdam ESHRE/ASRM-Sponsored 3rd PCOS Consensus Workshop Group. Hum Reprod. 2012;**27**:14–24.

5. Morley LC, Tang T, Yasmin E, Norman RJ, Balen AH. Insulin-sensitising drugs (metformin, rosiglitazone, pioglitazone, D-chiro-inositol) for women with polycystic ovary syndrome, oligo amenorrhoea and subfertility. Cochrane Database Syst Rev. 2017;**11**:CD003053.

6. Harper J, Boivin J, O'Neill HC, Brian K, Dhingra J, Dugdale G, et al. The need to improve fertility awareness. Reprod Biomed Online. 2017;**4**:18–20.

7. Wijeyeratne C, Udayangani D, Balen AH. Ethnic specific PCOS. Exp Rev Endocrinol Metabol. 2013;**8**:71–9.

8. Balen AH, Morley LC, Misso M, Franks S, Legro RS, Wijeyaratne CN, et al. WHO recommendations for the management of anovulatory infertility in women with polycystic ovary syndrome (PCOS). Hum Reprod Update. 2016;**22**:687–708.

Müllerian Duct Anomalies

Cara E. Williams

7.1 Introduction

Congenital Müllerian anomalies occur in approximately 5% of females. Patients with simple anomalies may be asymptomatic and diagnosed incidentally during investigations for other gynaecological problems or in pregnancy. Others can present in a number of different ways and at different ages depending on the type of anomaly. The most common presentations include primary amenorrhoea, obstructed menstruation, dysmenorrhoea, dyspareunia, difficulty with tampons, infertility and recurrent miscarriage.

Clinical assessment, pelvic ultrasound and magnetic resonance imaging are all useful for investigating anomalies of the Müllerian tract. Trans-vaginal ultrasound is less useful in adolescent girls who may never have been sexually active or may not have a vagina. In these cases and also for more complex anomalies requiring detailed preoperative planning, magnetic resonance imaging (MRI) should be used. This has been found to correlate very well with clinical findings when assessing Müllerian and vaginal anomalies.

Complex Müllerian anomalies should be discussed in a multidisciplinary team comprising specialist gynaecologists, urologists, clinical nurse specialists, radiologists and psychologists. This is an NHS England recommendation for congenital gynaecological anomalies.

There are various different classification systems for Müllerian anomalies, with the most widely used being the American Society of Reproductive Medicine classification [1]. However, this classification system does not describe the vaginal anomalies well. The European Society of Human Reproduction and Embryology (ESHRE) and the European Society for Gynaecological Endoscopy (ESGE) have developed a newer classification system for Müllerian anomalies [2]. This categorises anomalies based on the anatomical variation with uterine, cervical and vaginal anomalies having independent subgroups.

Müllerian anomalies are frequently associated with renal malformations due to their common embryological development and imaging of the renal tract should be performed in all cases.

7.2 Embryology

An understanding of the development of the Müllerian duct is essential for the diagnosis and management of Müllerian anomalies. Undifferentiated ducts (Müllerian and Wolffian) begin to develop during the sixth week of embryonic development. In the absence of an SRY gene and therefore no anti-Müllerian hormone, the Müllerian ducts continue to develop caudally and medially with midline fusion to create the fallopian tubes, uterus, cervix and upper vagina.

The urogenital sinus forms by week 7. Cells proliferate from the upper portion of the urogenital sinus to form structures called the sinovaginal bulbs. These fuse to form the vaginal plate, which extends from the Müllerian ducts to the urogenital sinus. This plate begins to canalise, starting at the hymen and proceeding upwards to the cervix. This process is complete by 21 weeks of gestation.

7.3 Imperforate Hymen

The hymen is a thin membrane which separates the vaginal lumen from the cavity of the urogenital sinus until late fetal life. It usually becomes perforate before or shortly after birth. The incidence of imperforate hymen is approximately 1:1000 live female births. Classic presentation is that of increasing cyclical pain in the absence of menstruation in adolescence. On clinical examination, there may be a palpable pelvic mass per abdomen or on ultrasound scan. On gently parting the labia, there may be a visible bulging membrane, with a bluish coloration due to the presence of blood in the vagina. Treatment is with incision, drainage of haematocolpos and resection of the hymen. If the hymen is not resected, there is a risk of re-obstruction. However, care must be taken not to resect too close to the vaginal mucosa, which may lead to scarring and stenosis at the vaginal introitus. Vaginal dilation is not usually required and long-term reproductive outcomes are good. Imperforate hymen are not associated with any other Müllerian duct or renal tract anomalies. See Figure 7.1.

7.4 Transverse Vaginal Septum

Transverse vaginal septae (TVS) are a rare type of Müllerian anomaly. The exact incidence is unknown but may be between 1:2100 and 1:72,000 [3]. They are thought to result from a failure of canalisation of the vaginal plate at the point where the urogenital sinus meets the Müllerian duct. Septa can be perforate or imperforate and vary in their thickness and location in the vagina. Imperforate septa present in adolescence with obstructed menstruation and haematocolpos. Girls with a perforate septum often have normal menses and usually present with difficulties with intercourse or tampons.

Transverse vaginal septa are classified according to their location in the vagina (low<3 cm from introitus, mid 3–6 cm, high >6 cm), thickness, and presence or absence of a perforation. Accurate classification using clinical examination, USS and MRI is imperative for planning treatment. Treatment involves surgical resection of the septum with anastomosis of the proximal and distal vaginas. It is important that the entire septum is resected to prevent vaginal stenosis and subsequent dyspareunia. Septa can be resected vaginally, laparoscopically or via an abdomino-perineal approach depending on the classification of the septum [3].

Thin (<1 cm) perforate septa can be operated on vaginally, with low complication rates and good long-term reproductive outcomes. Occasionally, rotation of perineal skin flaps is required to bridge the vaginal defect and ensure a normal calibre vagina. Septa that are mid or high and <2 cm thick with an adequately distended proximal vagina and no other complex pelvic anomalies are suitable for laparoscopic resection [4]. These have also been shown to have low complication rates and good long-term reproductive outcomes. More complex septa (>2 cm thick, imperforate septae) will require an abdomino-perineal approach, due to the possibility that a bowel segment may be required to bridge the gap between the proximal and distal vaginas. Skin grafts have also been used for this purpose, but these are often unsuccessful when there is scarring from previous

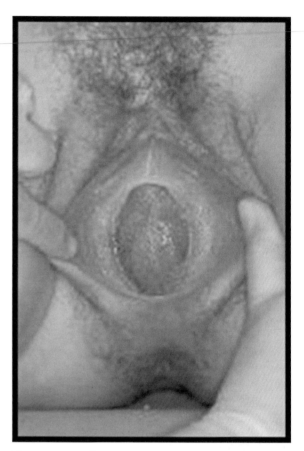

Figure 7.1 Imperforate hymen.

surgery, and there is a risk of scarring and vaginal stenosis in the donor region. More recently buccal mucosa has also been used to bridge the gap between the proximal and distal vaginas. Abdomino-perineal vaginoplasties often involve complex reconstructive surgery and therefore long-term complications such as re-obstruction and fistulae are more common [3].

Vaginal dilation is recommended following all laparoscopic and abdomino-perineal vaginoplasties, and where rotational skin flaps are used in vaginal resection. This helps to maintain vaginal capacity and prevent stenosis or re-obstruction, although there is little evidence-base to support this. See Figure 7.2.

7.5 Longitudinal Vaginal Septum

Longitudinal vaginal septa result from a failure of canalisation of the vaginal plate during embryogenesis. Septa can be complete, extending from the cervix to the introitus, or they can be partial involving any part of the vagina. They often present with dyspareunia or difficulty inserting tampons, or they may even be diagnosed during labour. Occasionally, one hemivagina may be obstructed resulting in regular menstruation with a history of gradually worsening pelvic pain, secondary to obstructed menstruation. Examination may reveal a unilateral vaginal wall swelling secondary to haematocolpos. MRI is the imaging modality of choice for these anomalies. In the majority of cases, there is an associated uterine anomaly, most commonly a complete uterine septum or uterus didelphys. Obstructed hemivaginas can be associated with renal anomalies on the same side as the obstruction, as in the OHVIRA (obstructed hemivagina and ipsilateral renal anomaly) syndrome.

Treatment usually involves surgical resection of the septum if the girl is symptomatic. The entire septum must be excised to avoid dyspareunia. This can be performed vaginally, with low complication rates and good long-term outcomes. Care must be taken with haemostasis due to the vascular nature of the vagina. Dilation is rarely required following surgical resection. Obstructed hemivaginas can be surgically more challenging, and therefore should be managed in a centre with expertise in operating on such anomalies.

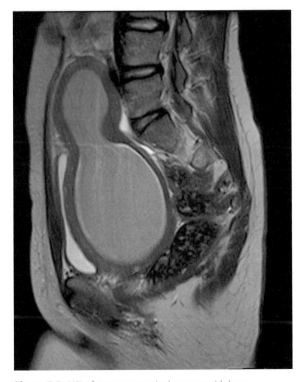

Figure 7.2 MRI of transverse vaginal septum with large haematocolpos and haematometra.

7.6 Uterine Anomalies

Uterine malformations account for the majority of Müllerian anomalies. They can be associated with recurrent pregnancy loss, infertility, preterm labour and malpresentation. The prevalence of uterine anomalies is approximately 5% in the general unselected population. This is not significantly increased in women with infertility (8.0%), but it is significantly increased in women with recurrent pregnancy loss (13.3%) and in women with infertility associated with recurrent pregnancy loss (24.5%) [5].

7.6.1 Arcuate Uterus

An arcuate uterus is characterised by a mild indentation of the endometrium at the fundus, less than 1 cm depth. The fundal contour is normal. This is a variant of normal and should not have any impact on fertility or pregnancy outcome.

7.6.2 Septate Uterus

Septate uterus is the most common congenital uterine anomaly (35% of all uterine anomalies). It occurs as a result of incomplete resorption of the septum following Müllerian duct fusion. These may be found during investigations for recurrent pregnancy loss or infertility, although they may also be an incidental finding in women with an uncomplicated obstetric history. The fibromuscular septa can be complete, extending from the fundus down to the cervix, or they can be partial, affecting any length of the uterine cavity.

An incidental finding of a septate uterus does not require surgical intervention in an adolescent. However, when a septum in found in association with infertility or recurrent pregnancy loss, then surgical resection via hysteroscopic metroplasty should be considered, especially if the woman is going to undergo assisted reproduction [6]. This has been found to be a safe and effective procedure. There are various different surgical techniques for resecting the uterine septum, but no particular technique has been found to be superior.

7.6.3 Bicornuate Uterus

Bicornuate uterus is a type of unification defect which accounts for 25% of uterine anomalies. It has been shown to be associated with an increased risk of miscarriage, preterm birth and malpresentation when compared with normal uteri and therefore pregnancy should be monitored accordingly. Surgery is not recommended if there is no obstruction to menstruation.

7.6.4 Uterus Didephys

Uterus didelphys is thought to account for approximately 10% of uterine anomalies. It is often associated with a longitudinal vaginal septum or even an obstructed hemivagina. Uterine surgery is not recommended, but an associated septum is likely to need resection. There is an association with renal anomalies including the OHVIRA syndrome as previously described. Imaging of the renal tract should always be performed.

Uterus didelphys is associated with a significantly increased risk of preterm and malpresentation when compared with normal uteri. There is a trend towards an increased risk of miscarriage but this is not statistically significant.

7.6.5 Unicornuate Uterus

Unicornuate uterus occurs when only one of the Müllerian ducts differentiates fully. When compared with normal uteri, unicornuate uteri are associated with an increased risk of miscarriage, preterm labour and malpresentation. Pregnancies should therefore be monitored accordingly.

There may be a rudimentary horn on the contralateral side which may or may not communicate with the normal side. If a non-communicating rudimentary horn contains functional endometrium, the girl will present with increasing abdominal pain with or without an abdominal mass. There is a potential for pregnancy to occur in these horns and therefore they should be resected; this can be done laparoscopically. Renal imaging is essential prior to surgery to identify any coexisting renal anomalies and identify the presence and course of the ureters.

Cornual ectopic pregnancies are pregnancies occurring in rudimentary horns. These can either be treated by fetocide and methotrexate or laparoscopy, although this is associated with a high risk of bleeding.

The long-term reproductive and obstetric outcomes in girls who have had a rudimentary horn removed are largely unknown, although there is a significant risk of preterm labour [7]. However, there are case reports of term pregnancies in this group [8]. If a non-communicating horn does not contain any functional endometrium and the girl is asymptomatic, the horn does not necessarily need removal.

7.7 Accessory and Cavitated Uterine Mass (ACUM)

This is a rare anomaly, characterised by the presence of an accessory cavity lined by functional endometrium, located in the myometrium of an otherwise normal uterus. Presentation is with chronic cyclical pelvic pain and severe dysmenorrhoea. Radiological expertise with ultrasound and MRI is required to diagnose and distinguish from a fibroid or adenomyoma. Treatment is with laparoscopic excision of the mass.

7.8 Cervical Agenesis

Congenital absence of the cervix is a very rare anomaly occurring in 1:80,000 to 1:100,000 births [9]. Presentation is usually with primary amenorrhoea and worsening lower abdominal pain, with or without a mass secondary to haematometra. It may be difficult to differentiate from a high transverse vaginal septum, and the diagnosis may only be made during definitive surgery. It has been shown to be associated with vaginal agenesis in almost 40% of cases [10].

Previously, treatment for cervical agenesis was a total hysterectomy. However, due to advances in assisted reproduction and laparoscopic surgery, first-line treatment is now laparoscopic utero-vaginal anastomosis. A uterine catheter is used to maintain patency and prevent re-stenosis. There have been spontaneous pregnancies following laparoscopic utero-vaginal anastomosis [11], but as this is a relatively recent treatment option in a young population, longer follow-up studies are required to assess the long-term reproductive outcomes. When there is associated vaginal agenesis management is more complex.

7.9 Mayer–Rokitansky–Küster–Hauser Syndrome

Mayer–Rokitansky–Küster–Hauser (MRKH) syndrome develops as a result of interrupted embryonic development and failure of fusion of the Müllerian ducts. It results in hypoplasia of the uterus and the upper two-thirds of the vagina. It affects approximately one in 4500 live female births. Ovarian function is usually normal therefore girls present during adolescence with primary amenorrhea in the presence of normal pubertal development and secondary sexual characteristics.

Diagnosis is usually by clinical assessment and pelvic ultrasound, although when there is diagnostic confusion, MRI may be required. Vaginal length can vary from a small dimple in the perineum to over 6 cm, although the majority will be <2 cm. Over 90% of patients will have rudimentary uterine buds although these are usually small and undifferentiated [12]. Very occasionally they can contain functioning endometrium resulting in cyclical pain, and these rudimentary uteri need laparoscopic resection. Although the ovaries function normally, they are often located ectopically and may not be seen easily on pelvic ultrasound. This has implications in both accurate and timely diagnosis and for fertility treatment.

The mainstay of treatment includes creation of a functional vagina, discussion around the issues of fertility including adoption and surrogacy, and psychological input. Vaginal dilation is the first-line management for creation of a vagina. Girls who are psychologically ready to dilate and are registered in a dedicated dilation programme with regular input from experienced clinical nurse specialists have over 85% success rates [13]. For those who are not successful with dilation, a vagina can be created through traction with a laparoscopic Vecchietti procedure.

Fertility options for women with MRKH include assisted reproduction with surrogacy, and adoption. Uterine transplantation is an exciting possibility for these patients but it is still in its infancy and some way off being offered as routine.

Key Learning Points

- Müllerian anomalies occur in approximately 5% of females, with common presentations including primary amenorrhoea, obstructed menstruation, dysmenorrhoea, dyspareunia, difficulty with tampons, infertility and recurrent miscarriage.
- If there is a blue bulge on vaginal examination, the diagnosis is an imperforate hymen, and this should be incised and excised. If there is no blue bulge, further detailed imaging with MRI should be performed to accurately define the Müllerian duct anomaly. Complex anomalies should be referred to a specialist unit.
- During the investigative work-up for Müllerian duct anomalies, menstrual suppression should be considered to alleviate symptoms.
- Always consider an obstructed Müllerian duct anomaly in the event of increasing cyclical pain even in the presence of normal periods.
- Resection of a uterine septum is not recommended in adolescence. It should only be considered when it is found in association with infertility or recurrent pregnancy loss, especially if the woman is going to undergo assisted conception.

References

1. American Fertility Society. The American Fertility Society classifications of adnexal adhesions, distal tubal occlusion secondary due to tubal ligation, tubal pregnancies, Müllerian anomalies and intrauterine adhesions. Fertil Steril. 1988;**49**:944–55.

2. Grimbizis GF, Gordts S, Di Spiezio Sardo A, Brucker S, De Angelis C, Gergolet M, et al. The ESHRE/ESGE consensus on the classification of female genital tract congenital anomalies. Hum Reprod. 2013;**28**(8):2032–44.

3. Williams CE, Nakhal RS, Hall-Craggs MA, Wood D, Cutner A, Pattison SH, et al. Transverse vaginal septae: management and long-term outcomes. Br J Obstet Gynaecol. 2014;**121**(13):1653–8.

4. Williams CE, Cutner A, Creighton SM. Laparoscopic management of high transverse vaginal septae: a case report. Gynecol Surg. 2013;**10**(3):189–91.

5. Chan YY, Jayaprakasan K, Zamora J, Thornton JG, Raine-Fenning N, Coomarasamy. The prevalence of congenital uterine anomalies in unselected and high-risk populations: a systematic review. Hum Reprod Update. 2011;**17**(6):761–71.

6. Homer H, Li TC, Cooke ID. The septate uterus: a review of management and reproductive outcome. Fertil Steril. 2000;**73**(1):1–14.

7. Pados G, Tsolakidis D, Athanatos D, Almaloglou K, Nikolaidis N, Tarlatzis B. Reproductive and obstetric outcome after laparoscopic excision of functional, non-communicating broadly attached rudimentary horn: a case series. Eur J Obstet Gynecol Reprod Biol. 2014;**182C**:33–37.

8. Adolph AJ, Gilliland GB. Fertility following laparoscopicremoval of rudimentary horn with an ectopic pregnancy. J Obstet Gynaecol Can. 2002;**24**(7):575–6.

9. Creighton SM, Davies MC, Cutner A. Laparoscopic management of cervical agenesis. Fertil Steril. 2006;**85**(5):1510.

10. Deffarges JV, Haddad B, Musset R, Paniel BJ. Uterovaginalanastomosis in women with uterine cervix

atresia: long term follow-up and reproductive performance – a study of 18 cases. Hum Reprod. 2001;**16**(8):1722–5.

11. Kriplani A, Kachhawa G, Awasthi D, Kulshrestha V. Laparoscopic-assisted uterovaginal anastomosis in congenital atresia of uterine cervix: follow-up study. J Minim Invasive Gynecol. 2012;**19**(4):477–84.

12. Hall-Craggs MA, Williams CE, Pattison SH, Kirkham AP, Creighton SM.

Mayer–Rokitansky–Kuster–Hauser syndrome: diagnosis with MR imaging. Radiology. 2013;**269** (3):787–92.

13. Ismail-Pratt IS, Bikoo M, Liao LM, ConwayGS, Creighton SM. Normalization of the vaginaby dilator treatment alone in completeandrogen insensitivity syndrome and Mayer–Rokitansky–Kuster–Hauser syndrome. Hum Reprod. 2007;**22** (7):2020–4.

Primary Amenorrhoea and Delayed Puberty

Elizabeth Burt and Ephia Yasmin

8.1 Introduction

Female puberty, driven by the hypothalamic–pituitary–ovarian axis (HPO), sees numerous alterations in the body secondary to the rise in oestradiol concentration. Whilst the onset, tempo and sequence will vary between individuals, delay in initiation of events or arrest during the process warrant medical attention. Pubertal transition requires not only an intact HPO axis but also functional reproductive organs.

8.2 Puberty and Its Delay

Female puberty is a slow linear process requiring approximately 3 years for completion. There is maturation of the HPO axis and subsequent coordinated hormonal patterns associated with ovulation and menstruation (Figure 8.1). Puberty is driven primarily

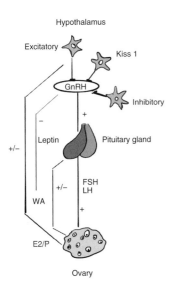

Figure 8.1 Hypothalamo–pituitary–ovarian axis.

by high oestradiol concentrations and culminates in the development of secondary sexual characteristics. Breast maturation and changes in bodily shape with growth and presence of axillary and pubic hair are the external phenotypic changes associated with puberty, whilst the attainment of an adult uterine configuration and many more subtle changes including those affecting the cardiovascular and neurological systems are internal alterations.

Puberty will start in 95% of girls between the ages of 8.5 and 13 years. Breast budding (thelarche) is usually the first sign of puberty and will begin in most girls by 11.3 years. Ninety-five per cent of girls will have achieved breast Tanner stage 2 by 13. The occurrence of menses occurs approximately 2 years after thelarche with an average age of 13 years. By the age of 14.5, 95% of girls will have periods [1]. The exact timing can be affected by multiple factors including ethnicity and BMI.

Primary amenorrhoea occurs in approximately 0.3% of females. Primary amenorrhoea with no secondary sexual characteristics by the age of 13 or in the presence of secondary sexual characteristics by 15 years of age is indicative of delayed puberty [1,2].

Some girls may already have a diagnosis with which pubertal development problems can be predicted, but for the majority pubertal delay may be first sign of an underlying issue triggering GP assessment.

Aberrations in the pubertal transition may be secondary to a spectrum of pathologies disrupting the HPO axis. If there is lack of both thelarche and menarche, this is indicative of complete early oestrogen deficiency. However, some may present with varying degrees of incomplete secondary sexual development suggesting an interruption at some point in the pubertal process. When primary amenorrhoea occurs in isolation and other secondary sexual characteristics are present this implies oestrogenisation and therefore alternative diagnoses should be considered as the cause is likely to be anatomical rather than hormonal.

Hypoestrogenaemia concurring with anatomical anomalies has been described, however this scenario is incredibly rare.

Puberty is a significant milestone in a girl's life and its absence will have not only physical but also psychological sequela. Lack of 'development' and not keeping up with peers can be highly distressing and this should not be forgotten nor overlooked in the assessment and treatment plan.

8.3 Causes of Primary Amenorrhoea

The aetiology of pubertal delay and primary amenorrhoea can be based on the presence or absence of secondary sexual characteristics (Table 8.1).

8.4 Absence of Secondary Sexual Characteristics

8.4.1 Constitutional Delay

Constitutional delay is a common cause of pubertal delay (14%) with overall delay in the maturation of the HPO axis. Usually other female family members will have experienced the same. There will be no other concerning features in the history and blood tests will reveal low gonadotrophins and oestradiol concentrations. All aspects of puberty will be delayed including growth velocity [3].

Although constitutional delay is considered a variant of normal, it can be clinically challenging

Table 8.1 Aetiology of pubertal delay and primary amenorrhoea based on the presence of secondary sexual characteristics.

Absence of secondary sexual characteristics	Presence of secondary sexual characteristics
Constitutional delay	Uterine outlet obstruction
Chronic illness	Mayer–Rokitansky–Küster–Hauser
Hypothalamic amenorrhoea	Polycystic ovary syndrome
Hypogonadotrophic hypogonadism	Hyperprolactinaemia and other endocrinopathies
Hypopituitarism	Complete androgen insensitivity syndrome
Premature ovarian Insufficiency	Pregnancy
Turner syndrome	
Swyer syndrome	

to differentiate it from idiopathic hypogonadotrophic hypogonadism, but in the latter there may not be a familial trend and there is ongoing linear growth without the pubertal growth spurt.

Treatment usually only involves reassurance and appropriate follow-up, but in some situations oestrogen induction of puberty may be necessary.

8.4.2 Chronic Illness

The mechanisms underpinning the pathogenesis of chronic illness and pubertal delay are multifactorial. Any chronic pathology either physical or psychological may be causative. Cystic fibrosis, chronic cardiac conditions, coeliac disease, emotional and physical abuse are just a few examples.

8.4.3 Hypothalamic Amenorrhoea

Hypothalamic function and GnRH pulsatility is sensitive to physical stressors such as extreme exercise, stress and calorific restriction leading to weight loss. The pathophysiology is thought to be mediated by leptin and depending on the timing of the insult, primary or secondary amenorrhoea may ensue. There is no particular threshold for the amount of exercise that will lead to amenorrhoea. The 'female athlete triad' is often coined whereby there is amenorrhoea associated with decreased energy intake and low bone density [4]. A BMI of at least $19 \, \text{kg/m}^2$ and a fat mass of 22% is thought to be critical for the onset of menses. Anorexia and bulimia, as well as other eating disorders such as orthorexia, may lead to amenorrhoea. Ultimately loss of hypothalamic drive will lead to hypogonadotrophic hypoestrogenic state and 3% of primary amenorrhoea cases are attributed to hypothalamic amenorrhoea [4,5].

Hypothalamic amenorrhoea should be a diagnosis of exclusion once all organic causes have been ruled out. Gonadotrophin levels may be normal/low with hypoestrogenic levels. Furthermore, blood tests may demonstrate hypercortisolaemia with hyperprolactinaemia and reduced IGF-1.

Although considered reversible if the underlying cause is eradicated, for example weight restoration, clinically there is often a lag between removing the trigger and resumption of GnRH pulsatility and gonadotrophin release. Indeed, in some, despite near normal gonadotrophin levels being seen, GnRH pulsatility is never repaired fully and some may remain amenorrhoeic and hypoestrogenic permanently.

Treatment is targeted at alleviating the underlying cause, but either temporary or more long-term, hormonal replacement may be required.

8.4.4 Hypogonadotrophic Hypogonadism

Hypogonadotrophic hypogonadism (HH) may be idiopathic but may be due to other acquired or congenital causes. Any physical destruction/compression of the central nervous system causes loss of GnRH/FSH and LH production. It may also be related to the production or functioning of GnRH at the genetic or molecular level. In addition to the amenorrhoea there may be related neurological symptoms including headache or visual field disturbance. Idiopathic HH may be reversible in some, but for most HH will be permanent [6].

Kallman syndrome is a rare (1:50,000) condition whereby there is defective GnRH neuronal migration to the arcuate nucleus. It is associated with colour-blindness and/or anosmia in combination with hypogonadism. Kallman syndrome may be sporadic in nature but may also have X-linked/autosomal dominant hereditary. One gene implicated is *KAL1*, which is essential for neuronal development.

Hypothalamic and/or pituitary function may be compromised or completely lost as a result of the mass effect of intracranial lesions such as craniopharyngiomas. Furthermore, the treatment of these tumours (surgical resection or adjuvant irradiation) can exacerbate the trauma to the area. Following radiotherapy, the gonadotrophic depletion may gradually develop several years after the initial insult. The hypothalamus and/or the pituitary may also be damaged secondary to head trauma or infections such as HIV or tuberculosis.

Whilst it may occur in isolation, HH can also be part of a more complex medical syndrome and primary amenorrhoea may be one feature of rare clinical spectrum syndromes including Prader–Willi syndrome, CHARGE syndrome or Dandy Walker syndrome.

Idiopathic hypogonadotrophic hypogonadism is identified when there is no underlying cause found and smell is normal. It may be very difficult to distinguish from constitutional delay of puberty. In some (10%–20%), reversal may occur, and therefore, once oestrogen therapy has achieved adequate pubertal and bone development, many advocate a trial off hormonal support to see if natural cycle resumption occurs.

8.4.5 Hypopituitarism

Global pituitary dysfunction with loss of the production and/or secretion of the pituitary hormones will lead to multiple comorbidities including hypogonadism. This may be congenital in origin in the case of septo-optic dysplasia or may be acquired secondary to tumours including pituitary adenoma, trauma, infection and inflammation. There will be other clinical and biochemical evidence of hypopituitarism.

8.4.6 Premature Ovarian Insufficiency (POI)

Premature ovarian insufficiency (POI) with hypergonadotrophic hypogonadism is defined as the loss of ovarian activity with amenorrhoea prior to the age of 40. Its incidence is quoted as 1% before the age of 40, but 0.01% prior to the age of 20. Therefore, primary amenorrhoea associated with premature ovarian insufficiency is rare, and secondary amenorrhoea is a far more frequent presentation. Often the cause of POI remains unknown, but autoimmune, genetic and infective origins have been implicated and need exclusion in the investigations. Iatrogenic POI may be secondary to gonadotoxic chemotherapy or radiotherapy [7].

8.4.7 Turner Syndrome

Turner syndrome (TS), with partial or complete loss of the X chromosome renders the ovarian follicular pool vulnerable to hastened atresia with varying degrees of preservation at the time of puberty. Five to twenty per cent will enter spontaneous puberty, but only 10% will progress through puberty, and most will experience pubertal delay and primary amenorrhoea. In addition to pubertal delay other stigmata of Turner syndrome may be present and require specialist investigation and monitoring including growth optimisation and cardiac health [8].

8.5 Presence of Secondary Sexual Characteristics

8.5.1 Müllerian Duct Anomaly

In the presence of a normal hormonal milieu and development of secondary sexual characteristics, primary amenorrhoea in isolation may suggest anatomical causes.

Uterine anomalies, also known as Müllerian duct anomalies, represent a spectrum of malformations seen in the female reproductive tract due to erroneous embryogenesis. The prevalence of uterine anomalies is approximately 5.5% in the general population. Despite their embryological origin, many are not detected until later in life due to an incidental finding or with the manifestation of their clinical sequela [9].

The Müllerian ducts undergo a series of complex transformations at approximately the sixth to eleventh week of gestation to form the uterus and upper two-thirds of the vagina. The external genital and lower portion of the vagina develop from the urogenital sinus. Uterine/vaginal anomalies may ensue secondary to problems with vertical or lateral duct fusion or defective resorption of the septum. There may even be complete agenesis.

Gynaecological and obstetric presentations may include primary amenorrhoea, irregular menses, dysmenorrhoea, endometrioses, pelvic pain, infertility, obstetric complications or sexual problems. Due to their shared embryological origins, uterine anomalies are also associated with renal anomalies.

MRKH, which affects 1 in 4500, is complete uterine agenesis. Due to an intact functional HPO axis, the classic presentation will be with primary amenorrhoea, normal gonadotrophins, presence of secondary characteristics and typically no cyclical pain. Less commonly, a rudimentary uterine horn with functional endometrium may persist. In this scenario the associated cyclical pain may confuse and delay the diagnosis. Whilst most cases are sporadic in nature there may be more rarely an autosomal dominant pattern. Ten to fifteen per cent of cases of primary amenorrhoea are thought to be caused by MRKH.

Outlet obstruction may be as a result of different anatomical variations including imperforate hymen, transverse vaginal septum (high, medium or low) or vaginal/cervical agenesis. Imperforate hymen is the most common (1:1000), whilst transverse vaginal septum has an incidence of 1:80,000. Presentation may be with primary amenorrhoea in combination with cyclical pain due to the accumulation of blood leading to haematocolpos and hematometra. Clinical examination may reveal the visible distinctive 'blueish' bulge of an imperforate hymen but may not detect any abnormality if the obstruction is high. Imaging in the form of high-resolution 3D ultrasound (US) or MRI is key to aid diagnosis, to locate the level of obstruction and any associated anomalies such as renal anomaly.

Treatment may render the primary amenorrhoea completely reversible in the example of surgical management of imperforate hymen/transverse septum.

8.5.2 Polycystic Ovary Syndrome (PCOS)

PCOS is associated with increased LH production, hyperandrogenaemia and disrupted folliculogenesis. PCOS is usually associated with secondary amenorrhoea but may, more rarely, present with primary amenorrhoea. In adolescents, ultrasound diagnosis is not recommended due to the high incidence of polycystic morphology in this age group. Diagnosis is based on the combination of amenorrhoea and hyperandrogenaemia (clinically and biochemically) [10].

8.5.3 Hyperprolactinaemia and Other Endocrinopathies

Elevated prolactin levels exert negative feedback at the level of the hypothalamus/pituitary with subsequent loss of FSH/LH secretion. This may be secondary to prolactinoma or medications. Symptoms and signs described may be associated with a space-occupying lesion itself such as headache and visual disturbance or may be secondary to the raised prolactin for example galactorrhoea.

Other endocrinopathies may interfere directly with pituitary function. Hypothyroidism leads to increased TSH levels which in turn stimulate both prolactin and FT4 release. Insulin is also known to mediate the HPO axis at multiple points and therefore insulin-dependent diabetes may also be associated with pubertal delay. Hyperandrogenaemia with excess testosterone levels may be secondary to androgen-secreting tumours, late-onset congenital adrenal hyperplasia and Cushing's syndrome and may lead to amenorrhoea.

8.5.4 Differences of Sex Development

Differences of sex development is a term encompassing many diagnoses where the 'development of chromosomal, gonadal and anatomic sex is atypical' [11].

The gonads remain undifferentiated until the seventh week of gestation. The Y chromosome houses the sex-determining region Y SRY gene, which is responsible for the differentiation of the gonad into a testis. In turn, the testes produce both anti-Müllerian hormone (AMH) and testosterone leading to the regression of the Müllerian ducts, persistence of the Wolffian structures and development of male external genitalia.

Primary amenorrhoea due to DSD may be secondary to either hormonal dysfunction or atypical anatomical development.

Swyer syndrome is a rare difference of sex development (DSD) affecting approximately 1 in 80,000 people. It is also known as complete XY gonadal dysgenesis. People with Swyer syndrome will have an XY karyotype but due to the gonadal dysgenesis and lack of AMH the Müllerian structures will persist and a uterus and upper 2/3 of vagina will develop. External genitalia will be of female phenotype. Multiple different gene mutations have been implicated in Swyer syndrome including SRY gene and the MAP3K1. Pubertal delay and primary amenorrhoea will manifest due to lack of hormonal drive and hypergonadotrophic/hypoestrogenic picture will be seen.

Androgen insensitivity syndrome (AIS) is another XY DSD secondary to an androgen receptor gene mutation. Its incidence is 2 to 5 per 100,000 and it has an X-linked recessive inheritance pattern, but may result from de nova mutations. Five per cent of cases of primary amenorrhoea are accounted for by AIS. Due to the presence of functioning testes there is regression of the Müllerian structures, but lack of receptor receptivity renders the testosterone inactive and external female genitalia develops. Sparse axillary and pubic hair and a short blind-ending vagina are characteristic. AIS may be complete or partial. With partial AIS there will be varying degrees of testosterone responsiveness and therefore virilisation, and those with partial AIS may present with atypical genitalia at birth. In contrast to Swyer syndrome, due to the aromatisation of the high levels of testosterone to oestradiol in the peripheral tissues, breast development and secondary sexual characteristics will develop but primary amenorrhoea will occur due to the absence of a uterus.

8.5.5 Pregnancy

Whilst usually presenting with secondary amenorrhoea and a 'missed period', in combination with other classic symptoms, pregnancy can often be overlooked as a less common cause of primary amenorrhoea and needs to be excluded.

8.6 Assessment

Assessment and initiation investigation should occur when there is

1. Primary amenorrhoea with no secondary sexual characteristics by the age of 13

2. Primary amenorrhoea in the presence of secondary sexual characteristics by the age of 15

3. Sooner, if combined with other symptoms/signs of growth delay, galactorrhoea, androgen excess, thyroid dysfunction or eating disorder.

The assessment and treatment are ideally carried out within a specialist multidisciplinary team with members providing expertise in paediatric gynaecology, endocrinology, psychology, radiology, urology and genetics.

In the knowledge that there may be many differential diagnoses of pubertal delay and primary amenorrhoea, having a clear systematic method to history taking and investigation is key. A thorough assessment is essential to ensure rapid and accurate diagnosis.

A sensitive approach, building rapport and signposting the expectations of the initial consultation including the need for personal questions is paramount. If attending with family, it is good practice to provide an opportunity to speak to the individual alone.

To facilitate diagnosis a suggested algorithm is displayed in Figure 8.2.

8.6.1 History Taking

The line of questioning will help determine which investigations to carry out. Specific questions should be asked, and some further clarification may be vital, for example referral may be due to 'primary amenorrhoea' but the individual may have experienced a small bleed sometime earlier that they did not feel 'relevant' to disclose. All causes of secondary amenorrhoea may also present with primary amenorrhoea, but secondary amenorrhoea excludes anatomical aetiology and indicates a previously intact HPO axis. Confusion may also arise when there is pubertal arrest as a small amount of breast development may be misinterpreted and labelled as the presence of secondary sexual characteristics.

Adolescence can be a particularly vulnerable time for many and understanding the dynamics and stressors is fundamental. Particularly relevant may be the family situation and progress at school.

Specific questions should include the following:

- Primary or secondary amenorrhoea
- Presence of secondary sexual characteristics (pubic and axillary hair and breast development) and timing

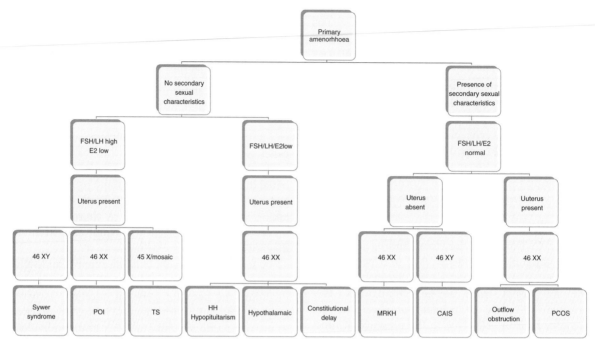

Figure 8.2 Primary amenorrhoea and delayed puberty.

- Associated symptoms such as pelvic abdominal pain (cyclical pain)
- Associated symptoms such as galactorrhoea/thyroid disease stigmata
- Neurological symptoms suggestive of space-occupying lesion – headache, visual field defect
- Anosmia
- Exercise pattern
- Calorific restriction
- Diet and eating trends, including previous significant fluctuations in weight
- Stress levels
- Sexual activity
- Previous medical and surgical history
- Medications
- Acne/hirsutism
- Family history of delayed puberty, premature menopause, fertility issues or autoimmune pathology
- School and family environment

8.6.2 Examination

At each consultation blood pressure, weight and height should be measured and body mass index (BMI)

calculated. A low BMI may indicate a hypothalamic cause. Short stature may suggest growth hormone deficiency associated with pituitary dysfunction or Turner syndrome. It is necessary to determine pubertal development using the Tanner stage.

With the advent of excellent imaging quality, genital examination, with its associated adverse psychological impact, is rarely justified in the clinical setting [12]. If indicated, genital examination should be performed under anaesthetic.

Neurological examination may also be necessary if there is any suggestion of space-occupying lesion.

8.6.3 Investigations

Investigations are required to establish the primary diagnosis, to investigate further the underlying aetiology and to provide information about treatment progression (Tables 8.2 and 8.3).

8.6.3.1 Blood Tests

Blood tests for gonadotrophins and oestradiol should be performed in all those presenting with pubertal delay and primary amenorrhoea. The pattern of results may point towards the cause and can be categorised based on the World Health Organization [13]:

- Group 1: Hypogonadotrophic hypogonadism (low FSH, low LH and low oestradiol) suggests hypothalamic/pituitary causes.
- Group 2: Normal gonadotrophins may be due to PCOS, anatomical or CAIS.
- Group 3: Hypergonadotrophic/hypogonadism (high FSH, high LH and low oestradiol) suggests gonadal causes.

Hormonal profile should also include blood tests for prolactin, IGF-1, thyroid function and testosterone. Prolactin levels greater than 1000 mIU/L warrant further endocrinology review and MRI assessment.

Table 8.2 Investigations for primary amenorrhoea

Investigations for all	Additional investigations that may be necessary
Gonadotrophins and oestradiol	Karyotype
Testosterone, SHBG and androstenedione	FRAXA screening
Renal profile	Autoantibodies
Prolactin and TFTS	MRI pituitary
Pregnancy test	MRI pelvis
Pelvic US	DEXA
	Tumour markers

Elevated testosterone levels may allow the differentiation between CAIS and MRKH when the uterus is absent on imaging. Anti-Müllerian hormone (AMH) is not useful for diagnostic purposes.

8.6.3.2 Imaging

Ultrasonography of the uterus is a non-invasive, well-tolerated, relatively fast imaging modality that has been used widely for pelvic evaluation. The uterus and ovaries are amenable to size and morphology assessment and pathology may be detected including hematometra/haematocolpus.

Ultrasonography should be completed by an experienced operator with an appreciation of uterine development and the ultrasound method should be considered to enhance image quality. In those who have been sexually active, a trans-vaginal approach may be used. The transabdominal approach employs the bladder as an acoustic window and therefore bladder filling needs to be optimal; however, image quality may be compromised due to body habitus. This may be circumvented by the use of a transrectal approach, which is a well-tolerated option with appropriate counselling.

Prior to oestrogenisation the uterus is small and tubular and in chronic hypoestrogenaemia the uterus may be too hypoplastic to be detected on both US and MRI. Therefore, caution should be exercised, as

Table 8.3 Diagnostic results associated with different diagnoses

	Secondary sexual characteristics	Gonadotrophins	Oestradiol	Ultrasound (uterus)	Karyotype
Constitutional delay	No	Low	Low	Small	46XX
Chronic illness	+/−	Low	Low	Small/normal	46XX
Hyperprolactinaemia	Yes	Low	Low	Small/normal	46XX
Hypogonadotrophic hypogonadism	No	Low	Low	Small	46XX
Hypothalamic	No	Low/normal	Low/normal	Small	46XX
Hypopituitarism	No	Low	Low	Small	46XX
POI	No	High	Low	Small	46 XX
TS	No	High	Low	Small	46X/mosaic/variation
Swyer syndrome	No	High	Low	Small	46 XY
PCOS	Yes	Normal	Normal	Normal	46 XX
Outflow obstruction	Yes	Normal	Normal	Haematocolpos/hematometra	46XX
MRKH	Yes	Normal	Normal	Absent	46 XX
CAIS	Yes	Normal	Normal	Absent	46 XY

although there are cases of Müllerian duct anomaly occurring in combination with hypoestrogenaemia, this is rare. Adequate oestrogen exposure (at least 6 months) should be given prior to making the diagnosis of uterine agenesis [12].

In addition to its diagnostic role, regular ultrasound assessment should be advocated during oestrogen replacement treatment to ensure adequate uterine development is achieved.

In certain situations, an MRI of the pelvis may be indicated. MRI may prove more beneficial when body habitus precludes adequate visualisation by US or when a Müllerian duct anomaly is suspected. MRI will allow delineation of anatomy for pre-surgical planning and provide further clarification of associated conditions such as renal tract anomaly.

An MRI of the pituitary may be necessary to exclude pituitary/hypothalamic pathology if symptoms or blood results are suggestive.

8.6.3.3 Genetic Testing

Karyotype analysis should be requested in those with raised gonadotrophins or an absent uterus. POI may be associated with genetic anomalies such as Turner syndrome and fragile X premutation. Balanced translocations of the X chromosome have been associated with amenorrhoea. Karyotype analysis may reveal XY karyotype suggestive of AIS or Swyer syndrome.

Although there may be a genetic origin for many other causes of primary amenorrhoea such as Kallman syndrome, until a single gene is identified, genetic testing is not useful. This may be an important discussion point in consultation.

8.6.3.4 Other Investigations

There is a panel of other investigations that should be performed depending on the clinical suspicion. A pregnancy test is necessary to exclude pregnancy in all those who have been sexually active.

In those with POI the detection of autoantibodies may suggest an autoimmune pathology and therefore blood tests for adrenal, thyroid and ovarian antibodies should be completed.

Oestrogen deprivation has a detrimental effect on bone health and therefore assessment of bone age/mineralisation depending on age, with hand X-ray or dual energy X-ray absorptiometry (DEXA), at diagnosis and during treatment is key to ensure adequate oestrogen replacement.

8.7 Treatment

The goals of treatment are multiple and should be considered within the multidisciplinary team at each review. Importantly what is considered the treatment priority for the clinician may be not be the same for the patient. Furthermore, the aims of treatment will change as the patient proceeds through 'life'.

Treatment aims depending on the underlying cause may include the following:

1. Pubertal induction with uterine and breast development
2. Bone health
3. Psychological
4. Fertility
5. Wider family implications/testing
6. Long-term HRT requirements
7. Restoration of anatomical function
8. Other surgical aspects, e.g. gonadectomy

8.7.1 Hormone Replacement

Timely referral and diagnosis ensure that the commencement of oestrogen treatment is not delayed in those who are hypoestrogenic. Induction of puberty aims to imitate spontaneous puberty over several years, with gradual exposure to exogenous oestrogen.

Transdermal preparations of 17β-oestradiol due to their physiological resemblance are favoured in the United Kingdom. Oestradiol delivered by the transdermal route does not undergo first-pass hepatic metabolism and therefore can be used in lower doses as there is no conversion to non-biological metabolites. Furthermore, by bypassing liver metabolism there are fewer effects on clotting factors and the production of other hepatic proteins.

Unopposed low-dose oestrogen should be commenced ideally between the ages of 11–12, although this of course will depend on the age of presentation. Titration of dosage to full adult replacement should be carried out over a 2- to 3-year window but the pace may need to be accelerated if the diagnosis is late. Although many protocols for artificial induction of puberty exist, the exact tempo of treatment should be individualised depending on the clinical response [1,8,14].

The aims for puberty induction are multifactorial and several endpoints should be used to assess the efficacy of treatment including hormonal profile, uterine dimensions, body shape, height, bone density and breast development.

Progesterone should be added to the regime to induce menarche (withdrawal bleed) after 2 years of unopposed oestrogen or to provide cycle regularity in those who have already experienced breakthrough bleeding. Establishment of regular bleeds is required for endometrial protection. The decision to add pro-gestogen is based on several considerations including duration of unopposed oestradiol, the presence of breakthrough bleeding, uterine size, endometrial thickness and breast development. It has been hypothesised that once progestogen is introduced, further uterine development is limited, and too rapid replacement could adversely affect the cosmetic appearances of the breast.

Long-term, optimal uterine development is essential for reproductive choice later in life as poor uterine growth has been associated with adverse reproductive and pregnancy outcome.

Adequate hormone replacement therapy (HRT) during the pubertal years and beyond, until the natural age of menopause, is crucial for long bone growth, bone mineralisation, cardiovascular health and general well-being and chronic oestrogen depletion is associated with osteopenia and osteoporosis. Vitamin D and calcium supplementations should be used in combination with oestrogen replacement for bone protection. HRT can be given in multiple preparations, but both oestrogen and progesterone are necessary for all those with a uterus. Preparations may be continuous combined or sequential depending on individual choice. Many opt to use the combined oral contraceptive pill (COCP) as this is felt to be more 'socially acceptable' as many peers will be using the same and can also provide contraception if required. To bypass the oestrogen-free week tricycling of COCP packs can be suggested. Reassurance as to the risks of HRT is necessary and women should be informed the risk of breast cancer with HRT is not increased before the natural age of menopause [7]. The risk of venous thromboembolism (VTE) in the context of COCP should be individualised and a transdermal preparation of HRT given if any personal history or risk factors for VTE.

8.7.2 Psychological

Emotional well-being is an essential part of patient care. Psychological sequela may stem from multiple sources. Insufficient pubertal development may lead to concerns as they fall 'behind' their peers. There may also be anxiety around disclosure, fertility difficulties and the stigma associated with chronic illness and long-term medication requirements.

Psychological input may be vital to reveal and tackle the underlying issues driving hypothalamic amenorrhoea such as distorted body image/obsessive behaviour and unhealthy eating patterns.

8.7.3 Surgery

Outlet obstruction may be amenable to surgical correction and ongoing anatomical patency with vaginal dilation will render the amenorrhoea reversible. Surgery varies in complexity and approach depending on the anatomy. Complex surgery should be carried out in a tertiary centre with the necessary experience and expertise.

Due to the risk of malignant transformation, prophylactic gonadectomy in those with XY DSD is current practice. Gonadal dysgenesis can give rise to gonadoblastoma, which in turn can progress to malignant germ cell tumours, the most common being dysgerminoma. The risk of malignancy is estimated to be between 15% and 35%. In Swyer syndrome gonadectomy is recommended at the time of diagnosis whilst in AIS later surgery is suggested, after the completion of puberty [11].

8.7.4 Fertility

Depending on the age of presentation, the fertility aspects may not seem 'significant' to the individual but providing the platform and opportunity for discussion pertaining to this should be promoted. The amount and pace at which information is given will be guided by the patient and clinical discretion.

Depending on the diagnosis spontaneous pregnancy may be a possibility. In POI a 5%–10% chance of spontaneous pregnancy is quoted and therefore contraceptive advice should be provided [7].

Depending on the underlying diagnoses, such as Turner syndrome, meticulous pre-pregnancy planning and health optimisation is crucial.

With an underlying pituitary/hypothalamic cause of primary amenorrhoea, pregnancy may be achieved in the form of assisted reproduction (ovulation induction or in vitro fertilisation, or IVF) by delivering exogenous gonadotrophins to stimulate ovarian activity and endometrial proliferation. In those who have no gonadal function, pregnancy using their own genetic gametes is usually not possible and options for fertility may include adoption or gamete donation.

Anatomical anomalies may preclude pregnancy, but ovarian function is still intact and therefore pregnancy may be achieved by the use of IVF in conjunction with surrogacy or uterine transplantation.

Key Learning Points

- There is a low threshold for assessment of pubertal delay +/− primary amenorrhoea to avoid diagnostic and treatment delay.
- Consider the possibility of both hormonal and anatomical pathology, depending on the presentation.
- Use of MDT is vital.
- Importance of psychological well-being should be considered.
- Hormone replacement for both pubertal induction and long-term health is recommended.

References

1. Conway G. Sex steroid treatment for pubertal induction and replacement in the adolescent girl. Scientific Impact Paper 40. London: Royal College of Obstetricians and Gynaecologists; 2013.

2. National Institute for Health and Care Excellence (NICE). Amenorrhea. https://cks.nice.org.uk/topics/amenorrhoea/management/2018.

3. Practice Committee of American Society for Reproductive Medicine. Current evaluation of amenorrhea. Fertil Steril. 2008;**90**(Suppl 5):S219–25.

4. Gordon C, Ackerman K, Berga S, Kaplan J, Mastorakos G, Misra M, et al. Functional hypothalamic amenorrhea: an Endocrine Society clinical practice guideline. J Clin Endocrinol Metab. 2017;**102**(5):1413–39.

5. Meczekalski B, Katulski K, Czyzyk A, Podfigurna-Stopa A, Maciejewska-Jeske M. Functional hypothalamic amenorrhea and its influence on women's health. J Endocrinol Invest. 2014;**37**(11):1049–56.

6. Viswanathan V, Eugster EA. Etiology and treatment of hypogonadism in adolescents. Pediatr Clin North Am. 2011;**58**(5):1181–20.

7. Webber L, Davies M, Anderson R, Bartlett J, Braat D, Cartwright B, et al. ESHRE guideline: management of women with premature ovarian insufficiency. Hum Reprod. 2016;**31**(5):926–37.

8. Gravholt CH, Andersen NH, Conway GS, Dekkers OM, Geffner ME, Klein KO, et al. Clinical practice guidelines for the care of girls and women with Turner syndrome: proceedings from the 2016 Cincinnati International Turner Syndrome Meeting. Eur J Endocrinol. 2017;**177**(3):G1–70.

9. Akhtar M, Saravelos S, Li T, Jayaprakasan K. Reproductive implications and management of congenital uterine anomalies. Scientific Impact Paper No. 62. BJOG. 2020;**127**(5):e1–13.

10. Teede HJ, Misso ML, Costello MF, Dokras A, Laven J, Moran L, et al. Recommendations from the international evidence-based guideline for the assessment and management of polycystic ovary syndrome. Fertil Steril. 2018;**110**(3):364–79.

11. King TF, Conway GS. Swyer syndrome. Curr Opin Endocrinol Diabetes Obes. 2014;**21**(6):504–10.

12. Ahmed SF, Achermann JC, Arlt W, Balen A, Conway GS, Edwards Z, et al. Society for Endocrinology UK guidance on the initial evaluation of an infant or an adolescent with a suspected disorder of sex development (revised 2015). Clin Endocrinol. 2016;**84**(5):771–88.

13. Rowe PJ, Comhaire FH, Hargreave TB, Mellows HJ. WHO manual for the standardized investigation and diagnosis of the infertile couple. Cambridge: Cambridge University Press; 1997.

14. Donaldson M, Kriström B, Ankarberg-Lindgren C, Verlinde S, van Alfen-van der Velden J, Gawlik A, et al. Optimal pubertal induction in girls with Turner syndrome using either oral or transdermal estradiol: a proposed modern strategy. Horm Res Paediatr. 2019;**91**(3):153–63.

Rokitansky Syndrome

Gail Busby

9.1 Introduction

Rokitansky syndrome, or Mayer–Rokitansky–Küster–Hauser syndrome (MRKH), also known as Müllerian agenesis, results from embryonic underdevelopment of the Müllerian duct, resulting in agenesis or atresia of the uterus, vagina or both. The vagina is shortened and may appear as just a dimple inferior to the urethra. A single midline uterine remnant may be present, or there may be uterine horns (with or without an endometrial cavity) which do not communicate with the vagina. This condition belongs to the most severe (class 5) of the ESHRE/ESGE classification [1].

9.2 Embryology

At around the fifth week of pregnancy, Müllerian ducts (paramesonephric ducts) appear. The caudal end of the ducts merge and become the superior two-thirds part of the vagina and uterine cervix, the intermediate part becomes the uterine body and the upper portions remain separate and form the fallopian tubes. In the same period the renal system develops, derived from Wolffian ducts (mesonephric ducts) within the mesenchyme of the metanephros.

Around this same period, there is migration of primordial germ cells from the yolk sac leading to the formation of the ovaries. These arise from mesenchyme and from the epithelium of the genital crest of the intermediate mesoderm. These processes are different and separate from those of the mesonephros, therefore anomalies of Müllerian ducts are not associated generally with anomalies of the ovary.

MRKH results due to failure of development between the fifth and sixth weeks of pregnancy and consequent fusion on the median line of Müllerian ducts, linked only to the caudal mesonephric ligament, destined to form the round ligament. The bladder and rudimentary vagina are unaffected as these arise from the Wolffian ducts and Gartner's duct, respectively [2].

9.3 Diagnosis

Patients with MRKH usually present with primary amenorrhoea with a normal female phenotype. Puberty is normal, with normal thelarche and adrenarche until periods fail to commence. On examination, patients with MRKH are normal in height, have normal breast development, normal pubic and axillary hair and normal female external genitalia. Vaginal examination reveals a shortened vagina, which may appear as a small dimple. There is no cervix at the apex of the vagina. See Figures 9.1 and 9.2.

Investigations reveal a normal 46XX female karyotype and normal sex hormone levels. Imaging reveals an absent uterus. There may be Müllerian remnants, either a midline uterine remnant or uterine horns, which may contain endometrium. The ovaries are,

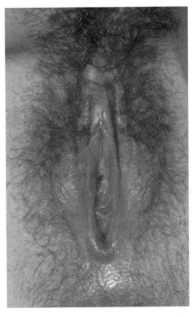

Figure 9.1 Examination showing normal external female genitalia. Note normal pubic hair distribution.

in the vast majority of cases, normal in structure and function, although they may be in atypical locations. Although a pelvic ultrasound scan is appropriate for initial imaging, magnetic resonance imaging (MRI) is the recommended imaging modality. Rudimentary Müllerian structures are found in 90% of patients with MRKH by MRI and this modality can also assess the presence or absence of endometrial tissue within the Müllerian structures. Due to the accuracy of MRI, there is no role for routine laparoscopy in the

diagnosis of MRKH. Some clinicians are content to use ultrasound as the primary imaging modality, reserving MRI for cases in which there is diagnostic uncertainty or pelvic pain. See Figure 9.3.

The differential diagnosis of MRKH includes obstructive uterine or vaginal anomalies and 46XY differences in sex development (e.g. complete androgen insensitivity syndrome). The former usually presents with painful primary amenorrhoea and a pelvic mass due to retained menses and the latter have sparse axillary and pubic hair and a 46XY karyotype.

9.4 Nomenclature

Rokitansky syndrome was first described by anatomist Bonn and physiologist Mayer in 1829 as a single case. Kussmaul (1859) and Rokitansky (1938) described one case each. Küster (1910) summarised the individual cases in a review paper of the literature, and finally Hauser named the 'rudimentary solid septate uterus with solid vagina' the Mayer–Rokitansky–Küster syndrome, to which his name was added, hence the name Mayer-Rokitansky-Küster–Hauser syndrome or MRKH.

9.5 Prevalence

The prevalence of MRKH has been estimated at 1 in 4000–5000 female births. A population-based study in Denmark, the largest to date, concluded that the incidence is 1 in 4962 live female births, in keeping with previous estimates. 168 patients were included, and patient characteristics described [3].

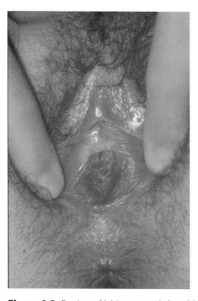

Figure 9.2 Parting of labia to reveal short blind-ended vagina.

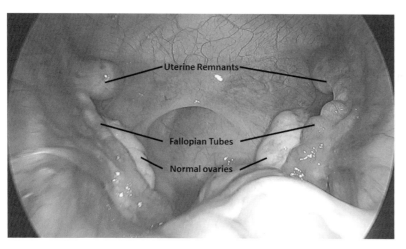

Figure 9.3 Laparoscopic view of patient with Rokitansky syndrome. Note normally sited and appearing ovaries bilaterally. The fallopian tubes are present, as are two uterine remnants.

Table 9.1 Types of MRKH

MRKH syndrome	Associated anomalies	Frequency (%)	
		Oppeit (2006)	Herlin (2016)
Typical	Tubes, ovaries, renal system normal	64	56.5
Atypical	Anamolies of ovary or renal system	24	43.5
MURCS	Anomalies in the skeleton and/or heart; muscular weakness, renal malformation	12	

Note. From Oppelt P, Renner SP, Kellermann A, Brucker S, Hauser GA, Ludwig KS, et al. Clinical aspects of Mayer–Rokitansky–Kuester–Hauser syndrome: recommendations for clinical diagnosis and staging. Hum Reprod. 2006;21(3):792–7; Herlin M, Bay Bjorn AM, Rasmussen M, Trolle B, Petersen MB. Prevalence and patient characteristics of Mayer–Rokitansky–Kuester–Hauser syndrome: a nationwide registry-based study. Hum Reprod. 2016;31(10):2384–90.

MRKH is divided into two groups: typical/type I (isolated utero-vaginal agenesis) and atypical/type II (associated with extragenital malformations of the kidneys, skeleton, heart and auditory systems). The most frequent of these are renal (34.2%), skeletal (12.5%) and cardiac (3.6%) This is in keeping with previous reports (see Table 9.1). Some cases of type II MRKH can further fulfil the criteria of Müllerian duct aplasia, renal aplasia and cervicothoracic somite dysplasia (MURCS). In this cohort, the distribution of typical MRKH syndrome was 56.5%, and that of atypical MRKH syndrome/MURCS was 43.5%.

Many extragenital manifestations have been described. Although not a completely exhaustive list, these are described in Table 9.2.

9.6 Genetics of MRKH

The aetiology of MRKH remains unclear. It is characterised by a heterogeneous aetiology and inheritance pattern. Familial as well as sporadic cases have been reported. Familial cases support an inherited predisposition, but a clear pattern of inheritance is yet to be described. The most frequent mode of inheritance appears to be autosomal dominant transmission with sex-linked (female) expression and incomplete penetrance. MRKH syndrome is, however, mainly sporadic [4].

Several gene mutations have been identified in MRKH patients including mutations affecting the following genes: LHX1, TBX6, WNT4, WNT7A, WNT9B.

Genetic counselling for families of patients with MRKH is complicated by the polygenic/multifactorial nature of inheritance. An empirical recurrence risk of 1%–5% has been defined for first-degree relatives.

Studies of the biological offspring of patients with MRKH via surrogacy have shown no affected babies reported, and only one male child with a middle ear defect.

9.7 Management Principles

The management of MRKH comprises three principles: creation of a vagina for coitus (if desired), fertility issues and psychological support. These management areas are all crucial for successful management of these patients, and therefore management should be within centres experienced in managing MRKH. These centres should possess a fully functioning multidisciplinary team able to offer a vaginal dilation programme, surgical treatment, fertility counselling, psychology and genetic counselling.

9.7.1 Vaginal Creation

Vaginal elongation is usually necessary in patients with MRKH for penetrative coitus to occur. This can be achieved by coital dilation (elongation of the vagina by repeated attempts at coitus), non-surgical vaginal dilation or surgical techniques of vaginal creation.

9.7.1.1 Primary Vaginal Dilation

Primary vaginal dilation is a non-surgical technique of vaginal elongation, originally described by Frank (1938), in which the vagina is lengthened and widened gradually using vaginal dilators of increasing lengths and widths being advanced via sustained, repeated pressure on the vaginal dimple until a vaginal length exceeding 6 cm is achieved. This technique has the advantages of being patient-controlled, safe, less painful and lower cost than operative techniques. This

Table 9.2 Extragenital malformations in MRKH

System	Frequency (%)	Anomaly
Renal	30–40	Unilateral renal agenesis (50%) Ectopia of one or both kidneys Renal hypoplasia Horseshoe kidney Hydronephrosis
Skeletal – spine	30–40	Scoliosis Isolated vertebral anomalies Klippel–Feil association Sprengel's deformity Rib malformation or agenesis Spina bifida
Skeletal – face and limb	16	Brachymesophalangy Ectrodactyly Duplicated thumb Absent radius Atro-digital dysplasia Facial asymmetry
Auditory	10–25	Middle ear malformations (stapedial ankyloses) Sensorineural defects Adysplasia of the auditory meatus

Note. From Morcel K, Camborieux L. Mayer–Rokitansky–Kuester–Hauser (MRKH) syndrome. Orphanet J Rare Dis. 2007;14(2):13.

technique was then modified by Ingram (1981) using a variation of the vaginal dilator and a bicycle seat stool. With this technique, the dilator is held in place by a light girdle, and clothing can be worn over this. The pressure is maintained for 2 hours per day by sitting on a specially modified bicycle seat stool. This avoids fatigue on the hands and the necessity to adopt lithotomy, squatting or Sims' position, and allows the patient to perform other activities during the hours of pressure required. Vaginal dilation via Frank's technique is still, however, the most frequently used method.

The most commonly reported reasons for discontinuing dilation prior to achieving success are lack of motivation and readiness. These issues should be explored prior to embarking on dilator therapy. The patient should be encouraged to start dilation when she truly feels ready and motivated to do so. Patients who start dilation prior to the age of 18 have lower anatomic success (47% vs 78%) when compared with those 18 and over, but both age ranges report similar functional success (78% in the under 18 group vs 76% of those 18 and over).

Other barriers to successful dilation include psychosocial issues (poor compliance, sociocultural factors, interpersonal conflict), cognitive issues (young age, lack of knowledge of process, underlying learning disability), logistical (lack of privacy, travel distance from clinic) and anatomic (discomfort/pain), scar from prior operation, absence of dimple [5].

9.7.1.1.1 Frequency of Dilation

In terms of achieving anatomical success, frequency may be more important than duration. Patients instructed to dilate for 10 minutes three times per day achieve higher rates of anatomic success when compared with those instructed to dilate once per day for 30 minutes (76% vs 46%, respectively). There is no difference, however, in functional success in these two groups (78% three times daily vs 84% once daily). Starting vaginal length is not correlated with ending vaginal length but may be associated with duration of dilator therapy.

Vaginal dilation can be associated with bleeding, pain or urinary symptoms. These can usually be successfully managed with appropriate support and advice. Thus, ongoing support during the dilation programme is paramount to success. This support is often nurse-led, with psychology input.

9.7.1.2 Surgical Neovagina Creation

The primary aim of surgery in the creation of a neovagina is to allow penetrative intercourse. There have been several techniques described, and no clear consensus exists regarding the best technique.

Regardless of the technique chosen, this should be performed by experienced operators as the first procedure is more likely to succeed than follow-up procedures.

9.7.1.2.1 Modified Abbe–McIndoe Operation

This procedure utilises a vaginal approach. A space between the bladder and rectum is dissected, a stent covered with a split-thickness skin graft is placed into the space, and vaginal dilation is performed postoperatively. There is a high rate of graft take and low rate of prolapse. Postoperative dilation is necessary and there is a high rate of graft contracture and neovaginal stenosis. Other issues include a lack of lubrication and a risk of squamous cell carcinoma. Complication rates are up to 14%. Modifications of this procedure include using allogenic tissue or autologous vaginal mucosa to line the neovagina.

9.7.1.2.2 Laparoscopic Vecchietti Procedure

This is a modification of the open procedure described in 1965 by Giuseppi Vecchietti. In the laparoscopic modification, the neovagina is created by internal upward traction on the vaginal dimple by an olive placed on the vaginal dimple which is attached to a traction device placed on the anterior abdominal wall. The olive is attached to the device by sutures which traverse the abdominal cavity. The traction device is tightened daily by 1 cm per day for 7–8 days until a vaginal length of 7–10 cm is achieved. The tightening of the traction device daily is painful and adequate pain relief is required. Postoperative vaginal dilation is also required to maintain the vaginal size unless regular coitus occurs. The benefits of this procedure are that it is minimally invasive, retains vaginal tissue and is not associated with excessive mucus production or vaginal stenosis. Vaginal dilation is necessary postoperatively and until regular coitus occurs. There is a risk of bladder or bowel injury when the traction threads are inserted. This procedure is not recommended in patients who have had previous surgery due to potential scarring as pliable tissues are required.

9.7.1.2.3 Laparoscopic Davydov Procedure

This procedure involves a laparoscopic and perineal step. The peritoneum over the vault is incised and the supravesical peritoneum is mobilised and a purse-string suture is placed at the level of the round ligaments and uterine remnants. The vaginal vestibule is then incised and dissection between the bladder and rectum is performed until the peritoneal edge is reached, which is then attached to the introitus. This is suitable for women who have had previous pelvic surgery, there is a lack of granulation tissue and no scar formation. The procure carries a risk of bladder or bowel injury, infection or prolapse.

9.7.1.2.4 Intestinal Vaginoplasty

This is the creation of a neovagina using a segment of intestine, most commonly a segment of distal sigmoid colon. The segment of bowel is isolated on its vascular pedicle and transposed down to the perineum. Ileum and jejunum may also be used. This procedure does not require postoperative vaginal dilation and can be performed in women who have had previous pelvic surgery. However, it usually requires a bowel anastomosis, can result in excessive vaginal discharge and carries with it a complication rate of 16%–28%, including postoperative ileus, bowel obstruction, diversion, ulcerative colitis and adenocarcinoma.

9.7.1.2.5 Williams Vulvovaginoplasty and Creatsas Modification

The Williams vulvovaginoplasty involves using full-thickness skin flaps from the labia majora, creating a neovaginal pouch. Vaginal dilation is then performed. The pouch is at an anatomically odd angle and the labia majora are hair-bearing skin, which will usually result in unacceptable cosmesis. This has been modified by Creatsas et al. This modification involves creating a pocket in the vulva by performing a U-shaped incision in the vulva, extending across the perineum and up the medial side of the labia to the level of the external urethral meatus. The inner skin margins are then closed, following which the subcutaneous fat and perineal muscles are approximated, and finally the external skin is closed. This procedure is associated with a 4% complication rate with wound opening. Patients can proceed directly to intercourse once healing has occurred without the need for vaginal dilation. Functional results are reported to be excellent but have not been subject to validated questionnaires.

The ACOG recommends vaginal dilation as first-line treatment for vaginal creation in MRKH [6]. A recent study showed that surgery is not superior to vaginal dilation in terms of global and sexual quality of life or anatomical results [7]. In this study, comparison was made between two groups of MRKH patients, one who had vaginal dilation and the other who had vaginoplasty by one of 5 different techniques. The majority of patients in the latter group had undergone sigmoid vaginoplasty (67%). Therefore, this study limits extrapolation to other surgical means of vaginal creation. Sigmoid vaginoplasty was also the major contributor to the 40% complication rate in the surgical vaginoplasty group.

9.7.1.2.6 Anatomical Success of Vaginal Creation Procedures

Anatomical success is defined as a vaginal length of at least 6 cm and the absence of complications associated with a cosmetically pleasing result (e.g. contractures, scarring). Non-surgical vaginal dilation is associated with normal vaginal lengths in at least 75% of women. Surgical vaginoplasty yields significantly higher anatomical success rates (>90% over 7 cm). In contrast, surgical vaginoplasty is associated with significantly higher complication rates than vaginal dilation [8].

9.7.1.2.7 Functional Success

Functional success is broadly defined as the ability to achieve satisfactory coital function. Using this definition, functional success from vaginal dilation is significantly lower when compared with vaginoplasty studies (74% vs 90%–96%). When functional success is defined as 'satisfaction with sex', however, the outcomes are similar (93% vs 96%).

The use of standardised questionnaires such as the Female Sexual Function Index (FSFI) [9] can assess female sexual well-being and provide a basis for comparison of functional success across the various techniques of non-surgical and surgical vaginal creation. This self-assessment questionnaire comprises 19 questions covering six domains of female sexual function: desire, arousal, lubrication, orgasm, satisfaction and pain. Scores range from 0–36.

Mean total FSFI scores in general reflect weaker functional scores after both vaginal dilation and vaginoplasty compared with the general population. Lower scores are evident in four of the six subscales: arousal, lubrication, orgasm and pain during intercourse. There are no differences for desire or satisfaction with sex life and/or relationships. No differences are found between different vaginoplasty methods, although numbers are small. Women who were treated with either dilation or vaginoplasty did not have better indicators of sexual wellness or sexual function

than those who were untreated, suggesting an important role of other factors beside treatment in these women.

In agreement with the ACOG, several other studies and reviews have advocated vaginal dilation, either by coitus or Frank's method as a first line in vaginal creation as it is less invasive and associated with much lower risk of complications with similar sexual outcomes as surgical methods of vaginal creation [10].

In the United Kingdom, vaginal dilation is the first line. In rare cases of unsuccessful dilation, the laparoscopic Vecchietti procedure is the surgical option of choice. It is noteworthy that, in the absence of regular coitus, regular vaginal dilation is required to maintain vaginal capacity.

9.7.2 Psychology

A range of reactions to a diagnosis of MRKH have been reported. These include depression, shock, fear of partner rejection and feeling different. Young women's sense of well-being and quality of life are impacted by a diagnosis of MRKH. These women will find it difficult, without treatment, to engage in penetrative intercourse, do not menstruate and will be unable to carry a pregnancy without major surgical intervention. These realisations can be devastating to an adolescent who has not yet achieved certain developmental milestones [11]. Patients have higher levels of anxiety and poorer mental health than normative data [12]. Women diagnosed with MRKH a mean of 10 years previously indicated scores for phobic anxiety, psychoticism and self-esteem that were between normal and psychiatric ranges [13]. This study also showed a similar trend to depression and anxiety. They also show higher scores on subscales Interoceptive Awareness, Interpersonal Distrust, Ineffectiveness and Bulimia.

The inability to carry a child has been suggested to be one of the most distressing effects of MRKH. This challenges women's self-esteem and gender identity and may lead to envy of peers who have children and a sense of exclusion.

The psychological distress around MRKH may vary over time, and it is thought that the most distressing time is soon after diagnosis. This is usually during adolescence at an important transitional life stage for identity formation and physical, cognitive and social changes. The severe distress which can be experienced at diagnosis may be alleviated by non-surgical or surgical treatment, the passage of time, counselling, parent support and group interventions.

Programmes offering psychological support for women with MRKH appear to be effective [14]. It is therefore important that psychological support is available at the time of diagnosis, and indeed throughout the life journey.

9.7.3 Fertility

In terms of achieving a family, if desired, women with Rokitansky syndrome have the following options: adoption, surrogacy and uterine transplantation.

9.7.3.1 Adoption

Adoption is an option which is devoid of medical intervention.

9.7.3.2 Surrogacy

Surrogacy is a fertility option in women with Rokitansky syndrome. This involves the patient undergoing IVF and the use of a gestational surrogate to carry the pregnancy and give birth to the baby. Surrogacy may be associated with religious and legal issues, making it a difficult or impossible option for many women worldwide. Regarding the reproductive potential of patients with MRKH, several issues may arise [15]. The first is the hormonal background of patients with MRKH. Several case reports and small cohort studies have reported that pituitary and steroid hormone levels are within normal limits. Also, 27 of 30 patients had normal anti-Müllerian hormone levels. This correlates with the clinical features of a normal karyotype, normally timed thelarche and pubarche, and evidence of ovulation.

Some patients had aberrant gonadotrophin levels, hyperprolactinaemia, high anti-Müllerian hormone (AMH) and hyperandrogenaemia. In a group of 69 women with MRKH, 60.8% had biochemical hyperandrogenaemia, but only a few had signs of androgen excess.

The second issue is the optimal ovarian stimulation protocol. In absence of menstruation, the menstrual phase determination is necessary in these patients to decide on beginning ovarian stimulation and synchronisation with the gestational surrogate. The combination of hormonal profile with ultrasound allows exact estimation of the patient's cycle phase.

A third issue is the technical feasibility of oocyte retrieval. In most reported cases, trans-vaginal oocyte retrieval is feasible. In some patients, this procedure may be difficult due to ovarian location (e.g. extrapelvic position). In these cases, transabdominal or transvesical aspiration have been used.

The age at which a woman undergoes assisted reproduction techniques (ART) is an important factor in fertility potential. Patients with MRKH seek treatment at a relatively young age as they have no alternative but to conceive via ART. In a systematic review of 14 reports of patients with MRKH treated with IVF and a gestational carrier, all the patients were under 37 years old. Patients' age influences outcomes in IVF cycles using gestational surrogacy in general.

9.7.3.3 Uterine Transplantation

Uterine transplantation affords women with absolute uterine factor infertility (AUFI) such as those with Rokitansky syndrome the possibility of carrying their own genetic offspring. Although there are other indications for uterine transplant such as hysterectomy for cervical cancer, postpartum haemorrhage and following unsuccessful myomectomy or for Asherman's syndrome, the majority of uterine transplants thus far have been performed in women with MRKH (88.9%).

The process of uterine transplantation involves first in vitro fertilisation 18 to 6 months before transplantation. Embryos obtained are frozen. The uterine transplant is performed and the patient placed on immunosuppression. The patient is followed up closely with gynaecological examinations, culture from the cervical canal and occasional cervical biopsies to diagnose infection or signs of rejection of the uterus. Blood pressure and body weight are also monitored along with serum creatinine, liver enzymes, blood count and iron stores, glucose and immunosuppressant levels. Embryo transfer is performed 1 year after transplant. During pregnancy, immunosuppression is continued and growth scans are performed. Delivery is by elective lower segment Caesarean section. Completion hysterectomy is performed after either one or two live births have been achieved. See Figure 9.4.

Eighty per cent of uterine transplants have been performed using live donors. The use of live donors allows benefits such as the ability to plan a complex operation requiring a highly skilled multidisciplinary team. It also allows time for counselling, assessment and investigation of the donor. Imaging of the vasculature of the donor uterus can also be undertaken [16].

The major disadvantage of use of a live donor is surgical risk. In the procedures performed to date, 11.1% donors experienced complications such as ureteric injuries (repaired intraoperatively), uterovaginal fistula and vaginal cuff dehiscence. Other

Uterine Transplant Timeline

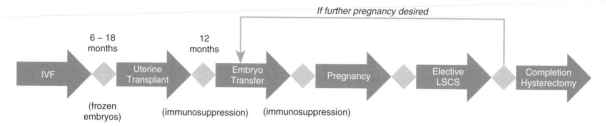

Figure 9.4 Rokitansky syndrome.

minor complications included wound infection, bladder hypotonia, urinary tract infection, constipation, leg/buttock pain, depression, intubation-related respiratory failure and anaemia.

There has been one live birth following donation after brainstem death (DBD). Although this avoids risk to the donor, it presents several logistical challenges. Transplant outcomes in general are superior in living donors, when compared with DBD, even when adjusted for differences in ischaemia times. Physiological optimisation and investigation of the donor organ is not possible with DBD. A significant issue also is the availability of appropriate uterine donors (i.e. female donors, between ages of 18–50, parous, uncomplicated obstetric history and lack of significant medical problems). It is expected that the number of fully eligible donors would be fewer than 50 women in the United Kingdom per year.

Most donor surgeries have been performed via laparotomy, but more recently, the robotic technique has been used.

More than 60 uterine transplants have been performed worldwide. A recent review summarised the outcomes of the 45 procedures on which detailed information is available: 13 (28.6%) have required emergency hysterectomy due to graft thrombosis (53.8%), infection (23.1%) or unspecified graft ischaemia (15.4%), and one (7.7%) was undertaken following postoperative haemorrhage. Other complications included 1 vesicovaginal fistula, 1 vaginal cuff dehiscence and vaginal stenosis which required stenting [4]. Five patients had minor complications such as urinary tract infections and postoperative pleural effusions. Seven women have had planned completion hysterectomies, 6 of whom had live births. Twenty-five (55.4%) continue to have functioning grafts [17].

During pregnancy, tacrolimus is used, either as monotherapy, or with azathioprine and/or prednisolone.

The first uterine transplant in humans was attempted unsuccessfully in 2000. This was a transplant from a live donor undergoing hysterectomy. Although cyclic proliferation of the endometrium with regular menses occurred for 2 months, the uterus needed to be removed 99 days postoperatively due to acute vascular thrombosis.

The second published uterine transplant occurred in 2011. This resulted in graft survival, permitting 2 embryo transfer cycles, both ending in early miscarriages.

In 2013, Brännström and his team conducted a clinical trial of 9 women undergoing uterine transplants from live donors. The results were 2 graft failures requiring hysterectomy and 7 graft survivals with subsequent delivery of 8 healthy babies [18].

In total, there have been 18 babies born to women who have undergone uterine transplantation, 17 from living donors and 1 from donation after brainstem death (DBD).

Uterine transplantation should still be considered experimental, although it is not unlikely that this modality of treatment may one day become mainstream.

All infants born following uterine transplantation have been healthy with no evidence of congenital malformations. Apgar scores at 10 minutes were normal in all offspring.

9.8 Gynaecologic Care

Health care providers should be sensitive to the fact that some routine gynaecological questions, e.g. the date of the last menstrual period, are unnecessary and can be distressing or result in a lack of confidence in the health care team. Similarly, due to the lack of a cervix, routine cervical cytology is not necessary. Routine pregnancy tests, for example prior to a surgical procedure, should be avoided.

The patient should, however, be asked about discharge, bleeding, pelvic pain and dyspareunia. Pelvic examination should be conducted if there are concerns about complications, vaginal stricture or stenosis, or if symptoms warrant this.

Sexually active women should be aware that they are at risk of sexually transmitted infections and condoms should be used for coitus. Human papillomavirus vaccination of girls and young women is recommended as it may decrease the risk of vulval and vaginal neoplasia and genital warts.

9.9 Conclusion

MRKH is a rare congenital anomaly of the female reproductive tract which requires a multidisciplinary approach. The diagnosis should be considered when a phenotypically normal adolescent female who has undergone an otherwise normal puberty presents with primary amenorrhoea. Diagnosis is by clinical examination, karyotyping, serum sex hormone levels and imaging. There is no role for routine laparoscopy in diagnosis as MRI is excellent at confirming the diagnosis. There is no single gene identified and, due to diverse genetic causes, genetic counselling can be challenging. Successful management comprises vaginal creation, fertility options and psychological support. These patients should be managed by an established multidisciplinary team. Vaginal dilation is recommended by the ACOG and many authors as a first line in vaginal creation, with surgical options reserved as a second line. Fertility options include adoption, surrogacy and uterine transplantation. Uterine transplantation should still be viewed as experimental, but worldwide experience with this procedure is increasing and this holds the promise of coming into mainstream use in the future.

Key Learning Points

- Rokitansky syndrome occurs in approximately 1:5000 female births.
- Diagnosis suggested by primary amenorrhoea after normal puberty, normal karyotype and short vagina and absent Müllerian structures on MR scan.
- Management principles include vaginal creation, fertility considerations and psychology.
- Patients should be managed by a multidisciplinary team experienced in the management of this condition.

- Uterine transplants are still experimental but hold the promise to become a mainstream procedure in the future for patients who choose this option.

References

1. Grimbizis GF, Gordts S, Di Spiezio Sardo A, Brucker S, De Angelis C, Gergolet M, et al. The ESHRE/ESGE consensus on the classification of female genital tract congenital anomalies. Hum Reprod. 2013;28:2032–44.

2. Pizzo A, Lagana AS, Sturlese E, Retto G, Retto A, De Dominici R, et al. Mayer–Rokitansky–Küster–Hauser syndrome: embryology, genetics and clinical and surgical treatment. ISRN Obstetr Gynaecol. 2013;2013:628717.

3. Herlin M, Bjorn AB, Rasmussen M, Trolle B, Peterson MB. Prevalence and patient characteristics of Mayer–Rokitansky–Küster–Hauser syndrome: a nationwide registry-based study. Hum Reprod. 2016;31:2384–90.

4. Fontana L, Gentilin B, Fedele L, Gernvasini C, Miozzo M. Genetics of Mayer–Rokitansky–Küster–Hauser (MRKH) syndrome. Clin Genet. 2017;91:233–46.

5. Oelschlager AA, Debiec K, Appelbaum H. Primary vaginal dilation for vaginal agenesis: strategies to anticipate challenges and optimize outcomes. Curr Opin Obstet Gynecol. 2016;28:345–9.

6. American College of Obstetricians and Gynaecologists. Müllerian agenesis: diagnosis, management, and treatment. ACOG Committee Opinion 728. Obstet Gynecol. 2018;131:e35–42.

7. Cheikhelard A, Bidet M, Baptiste A, Viaud M, Fagot C, Khen-Dunlop N, et al. Surgery is not superior to dilation for the management of vaginal agenesis in Mayer–Rokitansky–Küster–Hauser syndrome: a multicentre comparative observational study in 131 patients. AJOG. 2018;219:281.

8. Callens N, De Cuypere G, De Suttter P, Monstrey S, Weyers S, Hoebeke P, et al. An update on surgical and non-surgical treatments for vaginal hypoplasia. Hum Reprod Update. 2014;20:775–801.

9. Rosen R, Brown C, Heiman J, Leiblum S, Meston C, Shabsigh R, et al. The Female Sexual Function Index (FSFI): a multidimensional self-report instrument for the assessment of female sexual function. J Sex Marital Ther. 2000;26:191–208.

10. Herlin M, Bjorn AB, Jorgensen LK, Trolle B, Petersen MB. Treatment of vaginal agenesis in Mayer–Rokitansky–Küster–Hauser syndrome in Denmark: a nationwide comparative study of anatomical outcome and complications. Fertil Steril. 2018;110:746–53.

11. Bean EJ, Mazur T, Robinson AD. Mayer–Rokitansky–Küster–Hauser syndrome: sexuality, psychological effects, and quality of life. J Pediatr Adolesc Gynecol. 2009;**22**:339–46.

12. Liao LM, Conway GS, Ismail-Pratt I, Bikoo M, Creighton SM. Emotional and sexual wellness and quality of life in women with Rokitansky syndrome. Am J Obstet Gynecol. 2011;**205**(2):117.

13. Heller-Boersma JG, Schmidt UH, Edmonds K. Psychological distress in women with uterovaginal agenesis (Mayer–Rokitansky–Küster–Hauser syndrome, MRKH). Psychosomatics. 2009;**50**:277–81.

14. Wagner A, Brucker SY, Ueding E, Grober-Gratz D, Simoes E, Rall K, et al. Treatment management during the adolescent transition period of girls and young women with Mayer–Rokitansky–Küster–Hauser syndrome (MRKHS): a systematic literature review. Opranet J Rare Dis. 2016;**11**:152.

15. Friedler S, Grin L, Liberti G, Saar-Ryss B, Rabinson Y, Meltzer S, et al. The reproductive potential of patients with Mayer–Rokitansky–Küster–Hauser syndrome using gestational surrogacy: a systematic review. Reprod Biomed Online. 2016;**32**:54–61.

16. Brännström M, Kahler PD, Greite MS, Molne J, Diaz-Garcia C, Tullius SG. Uterus transplantation: a rapidly expanding field. Transplantation. 2018;**102**:569–77.

17. Jones BP, Saso S, Bracewell-Milnes T, Thum M-Y, Nicopoullos J, Diaz-Garcia C, et al. Human uterine transplantation: a review of outcomes from the first 45 cases. BJOG. 2019;**126**:1310–9.

18. Brännström M, Johannesson L, Bokström H, Kvarnstrom N, Molne J, Dahm-Kahler P, et al. Livebirth after uterus transplantation. Lancet. 2015;**385**:607–16.

Chapter 10

Turner Syndrome

Helen E. Turner and Matilde Calanchini

10.1 Incidence and Chromosome Abnormalities

10.1.1 Incidence

Turner Syndrome (TS) is one of the most common sex chromosomal abnormalities, caused by complete or partial absence of one X chromosome in a phenotypic female. The most common features of TS are short stature and premature ovarian insufficiency, but the phenotypic spectrum is widely variable in both presentation and severity.

The incidence is approximately 1 in 2000 live-born females, while analysis of cytogenetic screening studies suggest that TS occurs in 1 in 200 gestations, but most are lost as early fetal miscarriage, commonly due to cardiovascular and lymphatic development abnormalities and other less-well-defined causes.

10.1.2 Chromosome Abnormalities

Approximately 45% of live-born TS patients have X chromosome monosomy, 45,X. Other karyotypes may include structural abnormalities of the X chromosome, such as deletions of the short arm and duplication of the long arm to form an isochromosome (isoXq), ring formation (rX) and deletion in the long or short arm (respectively, Xq and Xp).

Mosaicism of a 45,X cell line with one or more additional cell lines, most commonly 45,X/46,XX, may occur (Table 10.1).

Approximately 10% of women with TS have Y chromosome material; they constitute a unique category because of their increased risk of developing a gonadoblastoma, a pre-malignant germ cell tumour with risk of malignant transformation. Reported rates of gonadoblastoma range from 2% to 50% and malignant transformation is rare, typically occurring after the second decade of life. Thus, the current recommendation is for laparoscopic, prophylactic gonadectomy [1], although there is little evidence about the appropriate timing for the procedure.

The phenotypic severity of TS is typically associated with karyotype, with in general the most severe phenotype occurring in women with 45,X monosomy and a milder phenotype in 45,X/46,XX mosaicism. However, the genetic basis linking the karyotype to phenotype is far from being elucidated. Comparative analysis of the karyotypes and phenotypes in TS is difficult, also due to the uncertainty regarding the extent of mosaicism in different tissues as the karyotype is usually based on a single examination of 30 peripheral blood cells. It has been hypothesised that all 45,X individuals who survive to birth have some degree of 'cryptic mosaicism' for a normal cell line somewhere in the body.

Table 10.1 Chromosome abnormalities in TS

	Karyotype	Frequency (%)
Monosomy X	45,X	40–50
Mosaicism	45,X/46,XX	15–25
Mosaicism with triple X	45,X/47,XXX – 45,X/46,XX/47,XXX	3
Isochromosome X	45,X/46,X,i(Xq) – 46,X,i(Xq)	10
Deletions	45,X/46,X,del(X) – 46,X,del(X)	6
Ring chromosomes	45,X/46,X,r(X)	3
Presence of Y material	45,X/46,XY – other with Y material	10–12

A number of pseudo-autosomal genes are present on the X and Y chromosomes that escape X inactivation and may be required in biallelic expression for normal development. So far, the only confirmed example of this genetic mechanism involved in the TS phenotype is short stature related to haploinsufficiency for the SHOX (short stature homebox) gene. Mutations and microdeletions of this locus result in short stature and some TS-associated skeletal anomalies.

Furthermore, preliminary studies suggest that the origin of TS-associated comorbidities may depend on a complex relationship between genes, transcriptional and epigenetic factors affecting gene expression across the genome.

10.2 Clinical Features and Diagnosis

10.2.1 Clinical Features

There is a wide variation of clinical features seen in females with TS, ranging from the severe phenotype with short stature, gonadal dysgenesis, characteristic dysmorphic features and cardiovascular congenital abnormalities, to women with only a mild reduction in final height and/or presentation with premature ovarian insufficiency.

10.2.1.1 Short Stature

Short stature is an almost invariable finding in women with TS. It begins prenatally, with poor growth often evident within the first 3 years of life. If left untreated, adult height is on average 20 cm below expected norms.

There is no evidence that growth hormone deficiency is a cause of short stature in TS, although partial growth hormone insensitivity may be a factor. Indeed, the recommended treatment during childhood consists of recombinant human growth hormone therapy in supraphysiological doses.

10.2.1.2 Bone Abnormalities

Many of the physical stigmata of TS (Table 10.2) are a result of structural bone defects, which rarely cause disability. Bone abnormalities include a shield chest with widely spaced nipples appearance, a short neck, cubitus valgus (increased carrying angle of the elbow), short metacarpals and metatarsals and Madelung deformity (bayonet deformity of the wrist). An increased risk of kyphosis and scoliosis is reported in patients with TS. The characteristic TS facies is

also primarily due to skeletal malformations. These result in micrognathia, a high arched palate and low-set ears.

10.2.1.3 Osteoporosis

The risk of low bone mineral density and fractures is increased in girls and women with TS. Several factors probably contribute to these findings, including inadequate oestrogen exposure and intrinsic bony abnormalities.

10.2.1.4 Other External Stigmata

Other specific features that might be present in a TS patient are pterygium colli (defined as webbed neck), irregular shape of the ears, low hairline at the back of the neck, ptosis, hypertelorism and epicanthal folds, and an increased number of melanocytic nevi (Table 10.2).

10.2.1.5 Premature Ovarian Insufficiency

TS is one of the most common causes of premature ovarian insufficiency failure. The gonads in TS differentiate normally until the third month of gestation, after which accelerated apoptosis of oocytes occurs along with an increase in ovarian stromal fibrosis. The pathogenesis of this process is yet to be

Table 10.2 External phenotypic features

Short stature	>95%
prominent epicanthic folds	20%
Epicanthus	10%
Ptosis	15%
Strabismus	
Ears	40%
Low set	35%
Irregular shape	
Micrognathia	60%
Abnormal dental development	70%
Neck	40%
Low posterior hairline	25%
Pterigium colli	
Thorax	30%
Broad chest	
Skin	25%
Lymphedema of hands and feet	25%
Multiple pigmented naevi	5%
Vitiligo	5%
Alopecia	
Bone abnormalities	50%
Cubitus valgus	35%
Short fourth metacarpal	10%
Scoliosis	5%
Madelung deformity	

determined. Pelvis ultrasound show that the majority of young TS have streak ovaries and, in many, the ovaries are too small to be identified. The uterus remains prepubertal in size if oestrogen treatment has not been started.

Approximately one-third of TS have spontaneous thelarche. Spontaneous menarche occurs in 5%–20%, most commonly in those having a mosaic karyotype. It is difficult to predict which girls with TS will have spontaneous menarche. Because of the ovarian insufficiency, many girls have elevated serum concentrations of follicle-stimulating hormone (FSH). However, measurement of anti-Müllerian hormone (AMH) may be more sensitive as a marker of pending ovarian failure than FSH [2].

Spontaneous pregnancy is rare and women with TS report infertility to be one of the greatest issues affecting their quality of life through all age groups [3]. Oocyte donation in vitro fertilisation (OD-IVF) and the recent techniques of fertility preservation increasingly offer the possibility of childbearing to TS women.

10.2.1.6 Cardiovascular Manifestations

Mortality is three-fold higher in TS women. TS-associated cardiovascular manifestations represent the most serious health problem for young and adult TS females and contribute to the increased morbidity and mortality seen in TS.

A bicuspid aortic valve is found in 30% of TS women compared with 1%–2% of the general population. This condition requires regular follow-up to exclude haemodynamically significant regurgitation and stenosis, where surgical intervention may be required.

Coarctation of the aorta is found in up to 17% compared with 0.04% in the general population. If left untreated, aortic coarctation may be complicated by severe hypertension, congestive heart failure and aortic dissection. It is commonly diagnosed during childhood when surgical intervention may be indicated.

Other congenital defects include elongated and kinked transverse aortic arch, aberrant right subclavian artery, partial anomalous pulmonary venous drainage, atrial and ventricular septal defects, and persistent left superior vena cava (Table 10.3) [4].

In addition to the congenital cardiovascular defects, hypertension is common in young and adult women with TS and is often independent of cardiac or renal abnormalities and of obesity. Loss of the nocturnal dip in blood pressure is commonly seen, and whilst current guidelines have no specific cut-off for treatment, it is reasonable to check 24-hour blood pressure values and have a lower threshold for intervention (e.g. >130/80 mmHg) if there are other cardiac risk factors. Some studies suggest that a general vasculopathy, as reflected by an increased arterial stiffness in TS compared with controls, might be a contributing factor. Cardiac conduction defects are also common and in particular prolongation of the QTc.

Aortic dilatation is reported in up to 30% of TS women and is associated with hypertension, bicuspid aortic valve and aortic coarctation, although it may also occur in the absence of these risk factors.

Importantly, aortic dissection affects 1%–2% of TS women and can be rapidly fatal if it is not promptly diagnosed and surgically treated. Risk factors for aortic dissection are the presence of hypertension, the presence of bicuspid aortic valve, aortic coarctation and aortic dilatation. In addition, pregnancy is a further risk factor due to the increased cardiac output. However, in 10% of TS who dissect no risk factors are identified. Aortic dissection is almost 100-fold higher than for women in general and is seen at a much younger age. Therefore, it is crucial to consider a diagnosis of aortic dissection in adult and young TS women with chest and back pain. The use of a wallet card to show to emergency personnel highlighting the risk/action for aortic dissection has proven helpful (Figure 10.1).

10.2.1.7 Renal Disorders

Congenital anomalies of the renal/urinary system affect 20%–40% of women with TS. The majority do not cause significant morbidity. The most common described abnormalities are horseshoe and partially or totally duplicated kidneys.

10.2.1.8 Hepatic Disease

Abnormal liver function tests are reported in more than 50% of TS women. Nodular regenerative hyperplasia and cirrhosis have been described, along with the more common condition of non-alcoholic fatty liver disease (NAFLD). Furthermore, biliary lesions, including bile duct paucity, biliary atresia, sclerosing cholangitis and primary biliary cirrhosis, are also more common in TS.

10.2.1.9 Autoimmune Disorders

TS is associated with an increased risk of developing autoimmune disorders, most commonly Hashimoto's thyroiditis (15%–30%) and coeliac disease (7%), but also inflammatory bowel diseases, diabetes mellitus type 1, alopecia areata, vitiligo, psoriasis and lichen sclerosus.

10.2.1.10 Metabolic Disorders

Patients with TS are at increased risk of central obesity, abnormalities in glucose homeostasis, including insulin resistance, decreased insulin secretion and overt type 2 diabetes mellitus, and dyslipidaemia. These conditions contribute to an already elevated cardiovascular risk.

10.2.1.11 Otological Disorders

Hearing loss associated with TS has several mechanisms. Conductive hearing loss consequent to recurrent otitis media is a problem in a significant proportion of children with TS. Progressive sensorineural hearing loss develops by adulthood in more than half of TS women, often requiring a hearing aid. An increased risk of cholesteatoma has been reported in TS.

10.2.1.12 Ophthalmic Disorders

Refractive errors are present in 40% of girls and women with TS, with increased prevalence of both hyperopia and myopia. Strabismus and amblyopia are more common and the prevalence of red-green colour-blindness is similar to that of males (8%).

10.2.1.13 Psychologic and Educational Issues

Intelligence is usually in the normal range, with the possible exception of individuals with ring X chromosome. Verbal skills are strong, while visuospatial awareness and problem-solving tasks might be more difficult. There is a reported increased risk of attention deficit disorder.

Studies on the incidence of psychosocial issues show conflicting results possibly due to selection bias and confounding factors such as short stature and infertility. No defined psychiatric condition has been traditionally related to TS, although conditions such as lower self-esteem and poorer psychosocial adaptation/interaction are often reported.

10.2.2 Diagnosis

TS is diagnosed at all ages, with peaks during fetal life, infancy, at prepuberty and early adulthood.

Table 10.3 Cardiovascular abnormalities

Cardiac congenital malformations	
Elongated transverse aortic arch	Up to 50%
Bicuspid aortic valve	Up to 30%
Aortic coarctation	Up to 17%
Pulmonary venous abnormalities	15%
Persistent left superior vena cava	10%
Atrial septal defects	2%
Ventricular septal defects	2%
Coronary arteries abnormalities	Up to 2%
Hypoplastic left heart	<1%
ECG abnormalities	
Prolonged QTc interval	Up to 35%
Hypertension	30%

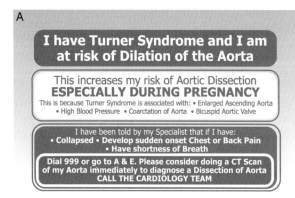
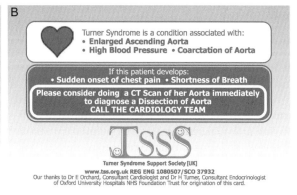

Figure 10.1 Cardiac alert card for aortic dissection in TS. Used with permission from the Turner Syndrome Support Society, UK, and available from https://tss.org.uk/information/healthcare.

In the newborn period lymphedema is the most common reason to screen for TS, whereas short stature, failure to thrive and less commonly cardiovascular abnormalities lead to evaluation during childhood.

Approximately 50% of cases are diagnosed later, typically as a teenager presenting with delayed puberty or primary amenorrhoea, and some even later in adulthood due to infertility.

Unfortunately, the highly varied phenotype causes not only diagnostic delay but also non-diagnosis. For example; delayed diagnosis of short stature is often associated with very little remaining potential for growth as later growth hormone therapy is associated with less catch-up growth. Early diagnosis also allows age-appropriate initiation of therapies for pubertal development in addition to timely screening, discussion and treatment for TS-associated abnormalities.

The diagnosis is made on the basis of a chromosomal analysis. A peripheral lymphocyte karyotype is routinely analysed and is diagnostic in the majority of cases. In rare instances, the karyotype is normal in females with TS mosaicism; however, if TS is suspected on clinical grounds, karyotyping of other tissue samples, such as skin fibroblasts, may be necessary.

10.3 Multidisciplinary Lifelong Management

Clinicians treating TS patients are challenged with many endocrine, genetic, cardiovascular, developmental, reproductive and psychosocial issues. Therefore, a TS-dedicated multidisciplinary approach to care is necessary and optimal.

Patient support organisations are also vital in providing support for TS patients as well as their family and partner [5].

10.3.1 Paediatric and Puberty

In childhood, girls with TS are monitored by a paediatric endocrinologist for screening for associated medical conditions and for initiation of growth hormone therapy, which can be started as early as 4–6 years of age. Careful follow-up during early childhood includes early evaluation and appropriate management of cardiovascular abnormalities, hearing impairment and refractive errors.

Due to early ovarian insufficiency, most girls with TS will not have spontaneous puberty and oestrogen replacement therapy to replace a deficient state is necessary for induction of puberty and for maintaining female secondary sex characteristics, normalising uterine growth and attaining peak bone mass. Studies suggest a positive effect of oestrogen hormone replacement on neurocognitive function and metabolic profile. Also, age-appropriate somatic sexual development has been associated with increased self-esteem and social development.

The aim of oestrogen replacement therapy in TS is to mimic the progression of puberty in the general female population. Annual measurement of serum FSH is suggested starting at the age of 10–11. More recent studies indicate that TS girls with low AMH are less likely to experience spontaneous puberty and menarche. Therefore, if there is no evidence of breast development, AMH levels are low and FSH levels are elevated, oestrogen replacement therapy should be initiated around the age of normal puberty (11–12 years). The initial dose of estradiol should be low in order to preserve height potential. Incremental dose increases should occur approximately at 6-month intervals to mimic the normal pubertal progression until adult dosing is reached over a period of 2–3 years. The primary consideration for a dose adjustment is clinical assessment, age and residual linear growth potential. If potential for taller stature is still possible (no evidence of epiphyseal fusion), lower oestrogen doses for a longer period might be considered.

Transdermal estradiol preparations are the preferred choice compared with oral oestrogens as they represent a more physiologic route of delivery, avoiding the hepatic first-pass metabolism. Estradiol is normally secreted into the systemic circulation and the liver receives the same concentration as other organs and tissues, whereas using oral oestrogen preparations, which are absorbed and metabolised by the liver, expose the liver to a greater concentration of oestrogen than the rest of the body. Accordingly, several studies highlight the advantages of transdermal estradiol preparations, including lower production of coagulation factors, lower risk for venous thromboembolism and the possibility to measure serum estradiol and guide sufficient dosage.

Progesterone should be delayed by at least 2 years to enable normal breast and uterine development or must be added once breakthrough bleeding occurs, due to the risk of endometrial cancer associated with prolonged unopposed oestrogen.

Once adult replacement doses are reached, treatment should persist until the average age of menopause. If there is significant bone loss, hormone replacement therapy may be continued longer after weighing up the risks and benefits of treatment. Notably, long-term hormone replacement treatment is not associated with an increased risk of breast cancer in TS.

10.3.2 Transition

The paediatric endocrinologist should plan a staged transition process to adult care in early adolescence evaluating the patient's readiness [1]. Joint paediatric – adult care programmes offer significant advantages for TS patients and their families. Early adolescence is ideally the time when paediatric and adolescent gynaecologists will start to be involved in the care of TS patients jointly with endocrinologists.

After the induction of puberty, the benefits of long-term oestrogen therapy should be discussed with each young TS girl, emphasising the importance for bone health and maintaining reproductive organ and psychosexual health.

Young women with TS are at increased cardiovascular risk; thus, promotion of healthy and active lifestyle, blood pressure monitoring and adherence to oestrogen therapy are key messages to be clearly discussed. If not previously performed, a complete cardiovascular screening is essential, including a thoracic magnetic resonance imaging to detect abnormalities that are more difficult to visualise with trans-thoracic echocardiography due to body habitus and the subjective nature of the technique.

Adolescence can be a particularly challenging period for a TS girl, and psychological, social and neurocognitive issues should be carefully considered during the transition period and appropriate counselling provided if needed.

Each young TS girl should be fully informed and counselled about the fertility issues, including emerging reproductive options such as fertility cryopreservation, the need for contraception and risks of pregnancy (see paragraph 4. Fertility, pregnancy and obstetric management).

10.3.3 Adult

Continued follow-up in adult TS is essential. Cross-sectional studies have shown that some TS-associated features become apparent in adulthood and/or are progressive with increasing age. Mortality in women with TS is three-fold higher than in the general population with the greatest excess mortality in older adulthood, and in particular increased mortality due to ischaemic heart disease and cerebrovascular disease. Many of the problems of adult life in TS women are compounded by obesity. Thus, lifestyle education must be included in a programme of prevention of hypertension, diabetes, dyslipidaemia and hepatic steatosis.

Selected parameters assessing health need to be repeated at intervals varying between 1 and 5 years, for example monitoring for aortic dilatation, metabolic conditions (monitor of HbA1 c and lipid profile), abnormal liver enzymes and autoimmune disease (including measurement of TSH, antithyroid peroxidase antibodies (AbTPO) and coeliac screening with tissue transglutaminase immunoglobulin A antibodies (AbtTG-IgA)) [1].

Screening for vitamin D deficiency is suggested and DXA scans to monitor bone density (BMD).

Key areas to cover are psychological and social issues, including relationships both personal and work related, sexual function and plans for future fertility. Sexual function should be specifically investigated as it may not be volunteered and women with TS might suffer from impaired sexual function. Referral to a gynaecologist with expertise in ovarian insufficiency in young women should be considered.

Additional aspects of TS that require regular follow-up are well described in published clinical guidelines [1]. From these guidelines it is clear that the long-term care of individuals with TS requires input from a variety of subspecialists. The best way to ensure that all recommended testing and management is appropriately performed is to use a standardised multidisciplinary approach. The use of an annual visit checklist for paediatric and adult TS patients is suggested (Figure 10.2).

10.4 Fertility, Pregnancy and Obstetric Management

10.4.1 Fertility

All adolescent and young TS women should be counselled that their probability to have a spontaneous pregnancy is rare, occurring in only 2%–8%, with the chances declining rapidly with age [6]. Predictors of spontaneous pregnancy include spontaneous

PAEDIATRIC HEALTH CHECKLIST

TURNER SYNDROME
TSSS
SUPPORT SOCIETY (UK)

Name:

Address:

Postcode:

Telephone: Mobile:

Date of birth: NHS No.:

Reference: Gravolt CH, Andersen NH, Conway GS et al. Clinical practice guidelines for the care of girls and women with Turner syndrome: proceedings from the 2016 Cincinnati International Turner Syndrome Meeting. Eur J Endocrinol 2017; 177(3):1-70.

DIAGNOSIS

TS DIAGNOSIS	Date	Age	How was TS diagnosed?	
Pre-natal				
Post-natal				

AT DIAGNOSIS		Date	Yes/No/Result
Karyotype			
Presence of Y chromosome			
Referral for gonadectomy			
Genetic counselling referral			
Cardiology referral			
Transthoracic echocardiography (TTE) and CT/cardiac magnetic resonance scan (CMR) for adolescents			
Hearing examination			
Ophthalmological examination			
Speech and language assessment Referral			
Pelvic and renal ultrasound			
TS Support Society information provided			
Cardiac Alert card provided			

MONITORING AND MANAGEMENT

GENERAL	Date	Date	Date
Check at each outpatient visit	Result	Result	Result
Height			
Weight/Body Mass Index			
Waist/hip ratio			
Blood pressure			
Check annually			
Thyroid function			
Glucose and HbA1c			
Bone age			
IGF-1			
Liver function tests from age 10 years			
Check 2-3 yearly			
Thyroid antibodies (TPO)			
Vitamin D			
Coeliac antibodies (TtG)			

As required		
Dietary and exercise advice	Clinical psychology referral	Dermatology referral
Hearing and ENT referral (yearly if concern)	Ophthalmology referral	Dental/orthodontic referral
Orthopaedic referral	Podiatry referral	Lymphoedema referral

GROWTH	Date	Date	Date
	Yes/No	Yes/No	Yes/No
Growth hormone treatment Name: Dose:			
IGF-1 measurement			
Check for scoliosis annually			
Growth hormone stopped			
Oxandrolone started			
Oxandrolone stopped			

PUBERTY	Date	Date	Date
	Yes/No	Yes/No	Yes/No
Spontaneous pubertal development Age:			
Breast development stage			
Spontaneous menarche			
Age:			
Puberty induced			
First period			
Low-dose oestrogen replacement Name: Dose:			
Breakthrough bleeding			
Progesterone Name: Dose:			
Counselling on role of oestrogen and bone health			
Sexual function, fertility/ cryopreservation discussion			

ACADEMIC/SOCIAL	Date	Date	Date
	Yes/No	Yes/No	Yes/No
Mainstream school			
Additional support required			
Neuropsychological assessment at key transitional stages			
HEEADSSS questionnaire:			
Home			
Education/employment			
Eating			
Activities			
Drugs			
Sexuality and			
Suicide/depression			
Safety			
Specific difficulties			

TRANSITION ACTIONS

TRANSITION TO ADULT CARE	Date	Date	Date
	Yes/No	Yes/No	Yes/No
Referral to adult endocrinologist/ gynaecologist with an interest in TS			
Specialist TS clinic referral			
Cardiology referral			
Gynaecology referral			
Fertility counselling			
Genetics referral			
Psychological support			

Post-growth hormone/pubertal induction assessment						
	Result	Date			Result	Date
Final height			Liver function			
Weight/BMI			Renal function			
Blood pressure			Vitamin D +/- bone density			
Thyroid function			Pelvic ultrasound (include uterine size)			
Thyroid antibodies (TPO)			Renal ultrasound			
Glucose/HbA1c			Echocardiogram/CMR			
			Bicuspid aortic valve			
			Aortic diameters			

June 2019

Figure 10.2 Visit checklist for paediatric and adult TS patients. Used with permission from the Turner Syndrome Support Society, UK, and available from https://tss.org.uk/information/healthcare.

ADULT HEALTH CHECKLIST

TURNER SYNDROME
TSSS
SUPPORT SOCIETY [UK]

Name:
Address:

Postcode:

Telephone: Mobile:

Date of birth: NHS No.:

Reference: Gravolt CH, Andersen NH, Conway GS *et al.* Clinical practice guidelines for the care of girls and women with Turner syndrome: proceedings from the 2016 Cincinnati International Turner Syndrome Meeting. Eur J Endocrinol 2017; 177(3):1-70.

DIAGNOSIS

TS DIAGNOSIS	Date	Age	How was TS diagnosed?
Pre-natal			
Post-natal			

AT DIAGNOSIS	Date	Yes/No/Result
Karyotype		
Presence of Y chromosome		
Referral for gonadectomy		
Genetic counselling referral		
Cardiology referral		
Transthoracic echocardiography (TTE) and CT/cardiac magnetic resonance scan (CMR) for adolescents		
Hearing examination		
Ophthalmological examination		
Pelvic and renal ultrasound		
TS Support Society information provided		
Cardiac Alert card provided		

MONITORING AND MANAGEMENT

GENERAL	Date	Date	Date
Check at each outpatient visit	Result	Result	Result
Weight/BMI			
Waist/hip ratio			
Blood pressure			
Check annually			
Thyroid function (TSH)			
Renal function			
Liver function +/- US/fibroscan			
Lipid profile			
HbA1c/Oral Glucose Tolerance Test			
Check 3-5 yearly			
Thyroid antibodies (TPO)			
Coeliac antibodies (TtG)			

HEART/BLOOD PRESSURE (refer to guidelines)		Date	Date	Date
	Review	Result	Result	Result
Blood pressure	Yearly			
Antihypertensive Name:				
Dose:				
Echocardiogram/CT Coarctation?	3-5 yearly			
Bicuspid aortic valve?				
Other anomalies?				
CMR and measurement (mm) or indexed for BSA of:	1-10 yearly according to risk			
Aortic arch (AA)				
Aortic sinus (ASI)				
Cardiology referral				

HORMONE REPLACEMENT THERAPY	Date	Date	Date
Each outpatient visit	Yes/No	Yes/No	Yes/No
Name:			
Dose:			
Check dose/route is optimal			
Vaginal oestrogen required Dose:			

FERTILITY AND REPRODUCTION		Date	Date	Date
	Review	Result	Result	Result
Sexual function	Yearly			
Pre-conception counselling	As required			
Fertility discussion +/- referral	Yearly			
Uterus ultrasound	Pre-pregnancy			
Cardiology review with pre-conceptual imaging of thoracic aorta and heart with TTE/CMR (see guidelines)	Pre- and post-pregnancy			

PREGNANCY	Date	Date	Date
	Yes/No/Result	Yes/No/Result	Yes/No/Result
Spontaneous/assisted			
Pre-conceptual referral for pregnancy management by multidisciplinary team with TS expertise (see guidelines)			
TTE pre-pregnancy, (review at 20 weeks gestation increase frequency if required – see guidelines)			
Blood pressure (review at each outpatient visit +/- treatment)			
Cardiac symptoms (review at each outpatient visit)			
Delivery plan (pre-pregnancy/ 1st visit/as required)			
Monitor as required:			
Thyroid			
Glucose			
Vitamin D			
TTE/CMR post-pregnancy			
Liver function tests			

HEARING		Date	Date	Date
	Review	Result	Result	Result
Hearing problems	Yearly			
Hearing test	1-5 yearly			
Hearing aid	As required			

BONE/SKIN		Date	Date	Date
	Review	Result	Result	Result
Bone protection	Yearly			
Fracture history	Each outpatient visit			
Bone density	3-5 yearly			
Spine T or Z score				
Hip T or Z score				
Naevus change	Yearly			

SOCIAL		Date	Date	Date
	Review	Result	Result	Result
Discuss home situation and relationships	Each outpatient visit			
Monitor employment status	Yearly			
Workplace stress	Each outpatient visit			
Mood assessment	Each outpatient visit			
Anxiety	Each outpatient visit			
Obsessive behaviour	Each outpatient visit			
Clinical psychology referral	As required			

Figure 10.2 (cont.)

menarche and mosaic karyotype 45,X/46,XX, although spontaneous pregnancy with livebirths has been reported in women with monosomy X. Thus, it is important to counsel all TS women about use of contraceptive methods to avoid unintended pregnancy.

The risk of miscarriages, most commonly early pregnancy loss, is significantly higher than in the general population. Chromosomal abnormalities in the offspring of TS women with spontaneous pregnancy and the possibility of prenatal genetic testing should also be discussed on an individual basis.

However, most women with TS will be infertile and this sensitive information should be shared in an open and early but developmentally appropriate manner. Importantly, the discussion about parenting choices (including adoption/surrogacy) and planning for fertility should be included and revisited at each annual visit of young TS patients.

Pregnancy may be achieved by oocyte donation and in vitro fertilisation (IVF). The pregnancy rate in women with TS who have had adequate oestrogen replacement therapy and endometrial preparation (endometrial thickness greater than 6.5 mm) is similar to that achieved in women with premature ovarian failure without TS, demonstrating the importance of early and sufficient oestrogen replacement [7].

Fertility preservation is potentially feasible in young TS. Oocyte cryopreservation after controlled ovarian hyper stimulation and the more invasive option of cryopreservation of ovarian tissue and immature oocytes are promising methods of fertility preservation [8,9]. Young TS girls and their families should be advised that fertility preservation in TS remains at an experimental level and is currently under intensive investigation with no reported successful pregnancies. Spontaneous onset of puberty, mosaicism and normal AMH and FSH levels for age and pubertal stage are important prognostic factors for cryopreservation in young TS girls and women. At present, fertility preservation before the age of 12 years is not recommended.

Adoption and/or using a gestational carrier (surrogacy) are also an option for TS women who desire to be parents, particularly if there is a high risk of maternal complications associated with the gravid stage. These options are important to discuss.

Spontaneous and assisted pregnancy in TS are both associated with an increased risk of complications [10,11]. The rate of early pregnancy loss is increased, as well the risk of pregnancy-induced hypertensive disorders, including pregnancy-induced hypertension and preeclampsia, and preterm delivery. The risk of maternal death during pregnancy and postpartum has been estimated to be as high as 2%, mainly related to aortic dissection. This risk is increased in multiple pregnancies, therefore only a single embryo transfer at a time is recommended. Whilst the recommendation of a single embryo transfer is routine in the United Kingdom, some women explore fertility treatment elsewhere with less stringent regulation. Thus education of the women is essential.

10.4.2 Pregnancy and Obstetric Management

The latest TS guidelines [1] offer recommendations on the prevention and management of maternal complications. All pregnancies should be followed by a multidisciplinary team, including high-risk pregnancy specialists, endocrinologists and cardiologists, generally at a tertiary care facility.

Prior to any pregnancy, women with TS should be counselled about both the high maternal risks associated with pregnancy, in particular focussing on the increased risk of aortic dissection, and the fetal risks of increased miscarriage, premature delivery and growth retardation.

Each TS woman should have a MRI of the thoracic aorta and heart performed less than 2 years before planned pregnancy. If aortic dilatation is present, particularly in association with risk factors for aortic dissection, including bicuspid aortic valve and aortic coarctation, avoidance of pregnancy should be considered. There is an ongoing debate regarding the aortic diameter above which pregnancy should be discouraged and further studies are needed [12]; however, it is clear that combined assessment with the cardiologist and maternal medicine specialist is essential before embarking on any pregnancy.

Prior to and during pregnancy blood pressure should be strictly controlled (135/85 mmHg) in all pregnant women and anti-hypertensive treatment promptly started if high blood pressure is found.

In addition, before contemplating pregnancy, each woman needs a complete medical evaluation, including echocardiography, ECG, monitoring of thyroid status and glucose tolerance.

Women with a risk factor for dissection should receive during pregnancy a close cardiac follow-up, including transthoracic echocardiography at 4- to 8-week intervals and in the postpartum period. Any evidence of aortic dilation may require cardiac MR (without gadolinium).

Vaginal delivery is a reasonable option in TS, although elective or emergency Caesarean section may be considered to reduce cardiac risk and to manage foeto-pelvic disproportion due to maternal short stature and narrow pelvis. A multidisciplinary plan for delivery should be made ideally by an experienced team in TS and/or aortopathy including obstetrician/maternal-fetal medicine specialist, cardiologist and anaesthetist [1].

Key Learning Points

- TS is caused by complete or partial absence of one X chromosome. Diagnosis is commonly made during infancy and prepuberty, although delayed diagnosis remains an ongoing problem, as it negatively impacts the management of many TS comorbidities, including effective treatment of short stature.
- TS is one of the most common causes of premature ovarian insufficiency. Long-term treatment with oestrogen-progestin therapy is essential to prevent adverse consequences of oestrogen deficiency.
- Congenital (e.g. bicuspid aortic valve, aortic coarctation) and non-congenital (e.g. hypertension, aortic dilatation) cardiovascular abnormalities represent the most serious health problems.
- Spontaneous pregnancy is rare. In vitro fertilisation with donor oocytes offers the opportunity to achieve pregnancy, although the maternal and fetal risks should be assessed before pregnancy. Follow-up by a TS-dedicated multidiscliplinary team pre, during and post pregnancy is required.
- Long-term monitoring of the different comorbidities associated with TS is crucial to improve the quality of life and reduce the increased mortality seen in TS.
  A multidisciplinary approach to care should be offered to young and adult TS women.

References

1. Gravholt CH, Andersen NH, Conway GS, Dekkers OM, Geffner ME, Klein KO, et al. Clinical practice guidelines for the care of girls and women with Turner syndrome: proceedings from the 2016 Cincinnati International Turner Syndrome Meeting. Eur J Endocrinol. 2017;**177**:1–70.

2. Hankus M, Soltysik K, Szeliga K, Antosz A, Drosdzol-Cop A, Wilk K, et al. Prediction of spontaneous puberty in Turner syndrome based on mid-childhood gonadotropin concentrations, karyotype, and ovary visualization: a longitudinal study. Horm Res Paediatr. 2018;**89**:90–7.

3. Sutton EJ, McInerney-Leo A, Bondy CA, Gollust SE, King D, Biesecker B. Turner syndrome: four challenges across the lifespan. Am J Med Genet A. 2005;**139**:57–66.

4. Mortensen KH, Andersen NH, Gravholt CH. Cardiovascular phenotype in Turner syndrome – integrating cardiology, genetics, and endocrinology. Endocrine Rev. 2012;**33**:677–714.

5. Turner Syndrome Society, www.tss.org.uk.

6. Bernard V, Donadille B, Zenaty D, Courtillot C, Salenave S, Brac de la Perrière A, et al. Spontaneous fertility and pregnancy outcomes amongst 480 women with Turner syndrome. Hum Reprod. 2016;**31**:782–8.

7. Chevalier N, Letur H, Lelannou D, Ohl J, Cornet D, Chalas-Boissonnas C, et al. Materno-fetal cardiovascular complications in Turner syndrome after oocyte donation: insufficient prepregnancy screening and pregnancy follow-up are associated with poor outcome. J Clin Endocrinol Metab. 2011;**96**:260–7.

8. Oktay K, Bedoschi G. Fertility preservation in girls with Turner syndrome: limitations, current success and future prospects. Fertil Steril. 2019;**111**:1124–6.

9. Mamsen LS, Charkiewicz K, Anderson RA, Telfer EE, McLaughlin M, Kelsey TW, et al. Characterization of follicles in girls and young women with Turner syndrome who underwent ovarian tissue cryopreservation. Fertil Steril. 2019;**111**:1217–25.

10. Hagman A, Loft A, Wennerholm UB, Pinborg A, Bergh C, Aittomäki K, et al. Obstetric and neonatal outcome after oocyte donation in 106 women with Turner syndrome: a Nordic cohort study. Hum Reprod. 2013;**28**:1598–609.

11. Bondy C. Pregnancy and cardiovascular risk for women with Turner syndrome. Womens Health. 2014;**10**:469–76.

12. Söderström-Anttila V, Pinborg A, Karnis MF, Reindollar RH, Paulson RJ. Should women with Turner syndrome be allowed to carry their own pregnancies? Fertil Steril. 2019;**112**:220–5.

Differences in Sex Development

Naomi S. Crouch

11.1 The Evolution of Differences in Sex Development

Differences in Sex Development (DSD) is an umbrella term which covers conditions arising from a difference in observed and expected sex development. This could include karyotype, gonadal tissue or genital appearance. Previously alternative terms were used, such as *intersex*, *pseudo-hermaphrodite* and *testicular feminisation*, but these were inaccurate and generally disliked by patients. A consensus was reached in 2006 to change the terminology to *disorders of sex development*, with individual conditions referred to by their genetic basis [1]. This has been largely accepted in the medical literature, with older more pejorative terms falling from use. Whilst more accurate, the term *DSD* has not been without its critics, and there is a move towards describing this group of conditions as *differences in* sex development, which would seem to fit more appropriately with the increased understanding in anatomical variance in those with no known medical condition. Similarly, where anatomical change exists, this is now referred to as showing *typical* or *atypical* anatomy. These terms will be used in this chapter. Individual conditions are referred to by their descriptions, such as 46XX or 46XY DSD, along with the underlying cause of the condition.

11.2 Prevalence

When the widest definition of DSD is applied the incidence is thought to be approximately 1 in 1000 live births, but this includes more frequently occurring conditions such as Turner syndrome, which is discussed in Chapter 10. For most individual DSD diagnoses, incidence is significantly rarer. Many conditions are autosomal recessive so a family history may be present, although many cases will arise due to new genetic mutations. Incidence is also therefore increased in communities where consanguinity is prevalent. DSD has a history long shrouded in secrecy and shame, so details may not be forthcoming, but enquiring gently about any older female relatives who were unable to have children may offer some suggestion of a DSD family history.

11.3 Presentation and Investigation

Many conditions, such as those which present with atypical genitalia will be apparent at birth. For those with 46XX DSD (congenital adrenal hyperplasia) babies may also present with a salt-wasting crisis in the first few days of life. This is most common in those who have been markedly virilised at birth and mistakenly assigned as a boy. Although the clitoris will be enlarged, labia majora fused and appear very scrotal in appearance, there will be no descended testes and should ring alarm bells for any examining paediatrician.

For those where a DSD is apparent at birth, care will be offered by a specialist DSD team, with local hospitals having a link to a tertiary centre. The core team will consist of a paediatric endocrinologist, psychologist, paediatric urologist and specialist paediatric nurses, with other members including a geneticist, biochemist, radiologist and gynaecologist as needed. International standards exist regarding investigations and expected standards of care [2,3].

However, many other conditions will not be diagnosed until adolescence and will either come to the attention of paediatric endocrinologists, with a failure to enter puberty, virilisation at puberty, or to gynaecologists, presenting with primary amenorrhoea. Again, care should be offered with a DSD team, with paediatric endocrinologists, psychologists, gynaecologists as the core members.

For adolescents initial assessment at presentation should include FSH, LH, E2, Prog, testosterone and karyotype. A pelvic ultrasound scan will identify the presence of a uterus or not and may be able to locate intra-abdominal gonads. However, it will not be able to confirm whether these are testes or ovaries, and girls and their parents should only be advised of this once all test results are back and a diagnosis is able to be confirmed. Where surgery for removal of gonads may be planned, an MRI would be the imaging modality of choice. This allows the gonads to be clearly identified, as they may be ectopically placed and lie anywhere in the line of descent.

Table 11.1 summarises the initial investigations and findings for those with the more common DSDs.

11.4 Diagnosis

Where a 46XY karyotype is present, it is likely either an interruption in the biosynthesis or action of

testosterone has occurred, or the gonads are dysgenetic. In either scenario, virilisation may or may not have occurred. For those with a 46XX with an atypical appearance to the genital area congenital adrenal hyperplasia (CAH) is the most likely cause, which is due to a block in the enzymes catalysing steroid development. This leads to an excess of androgens, causing intrauterine virilisation of a female baby. Figure 11.1 shows the pathways of testosterone synthesis, along with the enzymes needed for each step. A deficiency in any enzyme will cause a block and affect the production of hormones further down the pathways.

Previously diagnoses were often evasive, resulting in many 46XY conditions, with virilisation being grouped under 'partial androgen insensitivity syndrome'. A contributory factor may have been girls

Table 11.1 Initial findings for DSD investigations

Karyotype	Condition	External female genital appearance	Internal gonads and structures	Androgens (female levels)
46 XX	CAH	Atypical	Ovaries, uterus, tubes and upper vagina	Raised
46 XY	CAIS	Typical	Testes	Raised
	17βHSD/5αRD	Atypical	Testes	Raised
	Pure gonadal dysgenesis	Typical	Dysgenetic testes, uterus, tubes and upper vagina	Normal

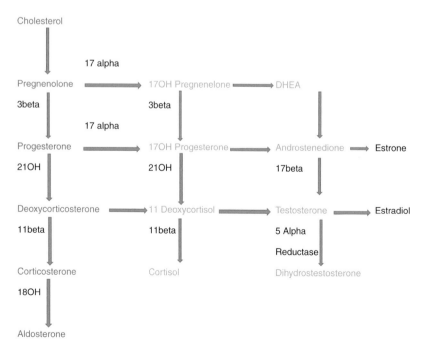

Figure 11.1 Testosterone and steroid biosynthetic pathway with enzymes shown.

having initial and limited investigations, with removal of gonads in hospitals which lacked extensive experience in DSD. The development of DSD services in tertiary care and the ability for rapid referral and review has minimised this, meaning all investigations and surgery will be under the care of a multidisciplinary team. Genetic studies have also developed rapidly over the last 20 years, allowing for the reliable diagnosis of many conditions, including those defects in the testosterone biosynthetic pathway. The net effect of these organisational and scientific advances is that girls and their families should have accurate diagnosis of their condition. The importance of this should not be underestimated. This allows understanding and explanations to be given, along with expectations for the future. It also allows access to peer support groups, and the option to take part in research studies. Finally, it also allows for genetic studies for unaffected family members, along with information on likely inheritability.

Once a clear diagnosis of a DSD has been made, it may be appropriate to offer screening to younger siblings in anticipation of other affected family members. Care should be taken with this, and involvement of an experienced DSD psychologist is mandatory.

11.5 Disclosure of Diagnosis

Historically the diagnosis of a DSD was rarely given or was clouded in inaccurate detail [4]. Women may have been advised that they had 'diseased ovaries' and needed an operation to remove them. Whilst this may have been with the best of protective intentions, this approach is inappropriate and deprives an individual of her medical information. It also does not allow for unaffected family members to have information on likely carrier status, and precludes any individual having the option to take part in research studies. More globally this leads to a lack of knowledge of long-term outcomes of treatments and health conditions, limiting information which can be offered to patients and parents of those who are newly diagnosed.

The overall effect of such an approach by clinicians was inadvertently to promote secrecy and shame and cast a stigma which is still felt by many patients. Medical details are of course always private, but are not shameful, and full disclosure of diagnosis must take place for any adolescent with a DSD.

This should be performed in a graded way, in conjunction with a psychologist. Timing will be individualised but generally would occur in mid-adolescence.

Information regarding previous treatments, methods of diagnosis, karyotype, potential for sexual function and pleasure, and fertility status must be fully covered so she ultimately has a full understanding of her medical condition. This would also involve working with parents to help support the process of discussing the diagnosis and dealing with questions as they arise, promoting a stance of appropriate privacy and understanding as opposed to secrecy and shame.

11.6 46XX DSD

Congenital Adrenal Hyperplasia (CAH), also known as 46XX DSD, is an autosomal recessive condition affecting 1:14,000 births. The commonest type of CAH is due to a lack of 21 hydroxylase, the enzyme catalysing conversion of the steroid pathway (see Figure 11.1). This leads to an excess of androgens in utero, which has the effect of virilising the female fetus. The clitoris is larger than usual, with the urethra opening near to the glans. The labia majora have a rugose appearance and may be fused. There is one single opening onto the perineum, with the vagina arising somewhere from the back of the urethra, internally. The appearance of the genital area is classified according to Prader stages, and is graded from 1 to 5 (Figure 11.2).

If CAH is not recognised at the time of birth a life-threatening salt-wasting crisis can occur due to a lack of cortisol. This represents a true medical emergency, in contrast to the differences in appearance to the genital area, which is an area for discussion with parents at a later time.

11.7 Management

Steroid replacement will usually be required, which must be carefully balanced with childhood growth. This should be under the auspices of a paediatric endocrinology team who are experienced in caring for those with CAH.

Historically, for those with atypical genitalia due to any underlying DSD diagnosis, feminising genitoplasty operations were performed in order to achieve a more typical female appearance [5]. This consists of separating and drawing down the vagina to open onto the perineum, reducing the size of the clitoris and trimming any excess labial or clitoral hood tissue. Various styles of surgery have been described over the years, but standard management would be a 'one-stage' procedure at a few months of age. However,

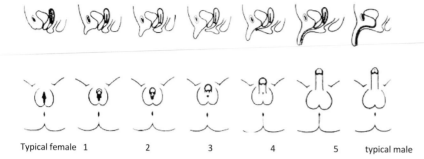

Figure 11.2 Prader stages to describe atypical genital appearance.

Typical female   1   2   3   4   5   typical male

despite the name, all surgery will require further revision at adolescence in order to allow tampon use and future penetrative sexual intercourse.

This approach to surgery has been challenged increasingly from many quarters. Children do not need a vagina, so to operate in infancy seems inappropriate when further adolescent intervention is indicated anyway. Clitoral reduction surgery is cosmetic. The clitoris has no other known function save for sexual pleasure, and an enlarged clitoris poses no health concerns for its owner. Surgery damages nerves and risks future sexual function [6,7]. Parents give consent for surgery under the age of 16, and therefore are being asked to agree to a procedure without medical necessity where their future adult children may hold an alternative view. Surgical outcomes on adults are limited, and those which exist show poor cosmesis and function, with 1:4 of those with clitoral surgery experiencing anorgasmia [8]. Adult gynaecologists and urologists have highlighted the need for continued surgical intervention despite 'one-stage' surgery having been performed. Increasingly vocal peer support groups have called for a review of surgery with some advocating a complete moratorium on all genital surgery until the child has capacity to consent as an individual. This is slowly being adopted by some regions and countries, with Malta and California now banning surgery, and the European Council issuing an advice document recommending the avoidance of any medically unnecessary surgery. However, worldwide early surgery in infancy remains the current standard practice.

Regardless whether surgery has occurred in childhood or not an assessment is offered at adolescence to ensure there is no obstruction to menstrual flow. Once this is assured, the timing of treatment to allow tampon use and penetrative intercourse can be deferred until a time of the individual's choosing.

11.8 46XY DSD

46 XY DSD can broadly be considered as either that which is due to some disruption in the biosynthesis of testosterone or gonadal dysgenesis.

The pathway from cholesterol to testosterone has many steps, with each being catalysed by a specific enzyme. Should this be missing, a block will occur with only partial virilisation occurring, for example 46XY 5 alpha reductase deficiency, or 46XY 17 beta dehydrogenase deficiency. For those where the pathway is intact, but there is a mutation in the androgen receptor itself, all hormone levels will be at normal male levels, but no virilisation will occur. This is known as complete androgen insensitivity syndrome (CAIS).

11.9 Complete Androgen Insensitivity Syndrome

Complete androgen insensitivity syndrome (CAIS) occurs in 1:40,000 births and is an autosomal recessive condition. It is rarely recognised at birth, as the external genitalia are typical for a female baby, with intra-abdominal gonads. These are normal functioning testes, and as such will have expressed anti-Müllerian hormone (AMH). This will suppress the Müllerian ducts and allow the Woolfian ducts to proliferate, resulting in no internal female structures such as uterus or upper vagina. The lower portion of the vagina is therefore shortened and blind-ending.

Girls may present with a hernia in childhood, which is the testis prolapsing into the labia. However, many others will not present until adolescent years, with primary amenorrhoea. Girls will also not have other signs of androgenisation, such as pubic or axillary hair, but will have normal breast development due to the peripheral conversion of androgens to oestrogen.

As height is carried on the Y chromosome, girls are often tall compared with normative female data. Whilst a diagnosis may be suspected with raised (normal male) testosterone levels, 46XY karyotype and an absence of internal female structures, this can now be confirmed in nearly all cases by identifying a mutation on the genes which code for the androgen receptor.

11.10 46XY Gonadal Dysgenesis

In contrast to CAIS, where the gonads are entirely normal, those with dysgenetic gonads will not have normal-functioning testes. This is either pure (sometimes known at Swyer's syndrome) or mixed gonadal dysgenesis. The testes will not have expressed AMH, resulting in internal female structures such as a uterus and upper vagina. The external genitalia will also be typically female. On occasion for those with mixed gonadal dysgenesis, low levels of testicular activity may occur, leading to reduced or no internal Müllerian structures. In this situation it is more likely the genital area will be atypical and the condition identified at birth.

For those with pure gonadal dysgenesis, the testes will also not start the pubertal process, so girls will present with primary amenorrhoea and no secondary sexual characteristics. With mixed gonadal dysgenesis some virilisation may occur, which could include voice deepening or clitoromegaly. Again, the Y chromosome will ensure that girls have a more typically male final height.

Table 11.1 shows a comparison of initial investigations and findings for the more common DSDs.

11.11 The Role of Gonadectomy

With CAIS the testes are entirely normal, although intra-abdominal testes do carry a small cancer risk. This is estimated at 5%, although data are flawed due to a historical lack of disclosure by doctors, meaning many women were unaware of their underlying condition [8]. Surveillance to detect precancer changes in the testes is problematic and currently not possible with imaging. For this reason, current practice is to retain the gonads until after puberty and then offer removal [9]. This means girls will need to take oestrogen-only hormone replacement therapy (HRT) until the age of the natural menopause. Some girls are

choosing to retain their gonads despite this, and careful counselling should be offered, with individuals aware of current limitations on health screening.

In contrast to the situation with CAIS, gonadal dysgenesis carries a 30%–40% chance of cancer development, and therefore gonadectomy is recommended at the time of diagnosis. HRT is indicated in any case for induction of puberty, and progesterone will need to be added once periods have established. This should be under the care of a specialist paediatric endocrinologist.

11.12 Psychology

An essential aspect of the care for those with DSD is support from a psychologist with specialist knowledge regarding DSD. Families and individuals will need time to understand a rare and complex diagnosis, and then in turn ensure full disclosure of details to the girl at the appropriate time. Girls themselves may have concerns about intimate examinations, potential future treatment and decisions regarding gonadectomy. In addition there is likely to be distress from the family regarding future fertility and paths to parenthood, alongside sexual function concerns. In contrast to often anticipated issues, the highest needs in adolescence are psychological, rather than medical or surgical, and these should be prioritised and met [10].

11.13 Long-Term Care Needs

11.13.1 Hormone Replacement Therapy

Where gonads have been removed, hormone replacement therapy (HRT) will be needed to provide oestrogen and prevent against osteoporosis. HRT is the best method to achieve this, with transdermal preparations preferred. In contrast to the oral contraceptive pill there is no increased risk in vascular events and replaces hormones to normative levels. Where a uterus is present progesterone will be required, which can either be cyclical or continuous, but otherwise HRT may be oestrogen-only. This should be continued until the age of the natural menopause. There is no increased breast cancer risk as HRT is restoring normal female levels of oestrogen rather than adding extra. Women may also require vaginal oestrogen, as younger women are more likely to be sexually active, and therefore symptomatic from local hypo-oestrogenisation. As part of monitoring adequate replacement, bone density measurements should be performed every 5 years or so, and additional measures advised if needed, to prevent against osteoporosis.

11.13.2   Fertility

For those with a DSD where a uterus is present, pregnancy is possible. Currently this would be with donated ova and an IVF cycle, but women are able to give birth normally and breastfeed. In UK law, the legal mother is the person who gave birth, rather than being genetically related, so no additional adoption process is needed.

For those without a uterus, options are more limited. Surrogacy represents the main way to have a baby, with a donated or the surrogate's ova, and again an IVF cycle. Non-commercial surrogacy is legal in the United Kingdom but remains a complex path, and for many is emotionally and financially challenging. In some countries commercial surrogacy is legal, where women are paid to carry pregnancies for couples. This is ethically challenging and also realistically puts this beyond the means of most. In contrast, surrogacy is illegal in many countries in the world, making access to parenthood via this method somewhat unequal worldwide.

Uterine transplantation may offer an option in the future for women with DSD with no uterus. However, this requires extensive surgery for both donor and recipient, and is still in the research stages.

11.13.3   Sexual Function

Many DSDs will have a shortened vagina as part of the condition. For women who wish to be sexually active and experience penetrative intercourse, vaginal treatment is likely to be required. Whilst many operations to create a new vagina have been described, the mainstay of treatment is the use of plastic dilators which are pressed against the vaginal dimple for approximately 30 minutes each day [11]. This has the effect of lengthening the vagina, and over 3–6 months will create a space suitable for intercourse. This has the advantage of avoiding any surgical risks, and also avoids scarring on the vaginal area, which can stenose and cause additional problems. Segments of bowel have been used previously, but this can cause excessive mucus formation, and also carries a cancer risk in the neovagina after many years. For this reason it has largely fallen from use.

Dilators are a straightforward, highly effective and low-resource solution for creating a lengthened vagina [12]. However, it takes a considerable amount of emotional resilience and maturity to perform this, and psychological support is mandatory. It takes time and is a reminder of a difference for the girl. It is important to reassure the girl that sexual pleasure, orgasm and intimacy are not dependent on having a vagina. Rather, this is related to clitoral function, and of course to relationship choices. For these reasons it is imperative that girls themselves choose when to start dilator therapy. It is entirely possible to have a happy and fulfilling life with a shorter-than-usual vagina, and therefore girls should not feel under any pressure to start treatment, although most women will choose at some stage to create a longer vagina.

11.13.4   Transition of Care

The vast majority of presentations of DSD will have paediatric specialists involved in care. However, those with DSD need lifelong care and arrangements must be made for transitioning care to adult services [13]. There is clear evidence from other chronic conditions that transition results in better outcomes for individuals, fewer emergency department presentations and increased engagement in health care. Transition is a process, as opposed to simple transfer of care, and takes place over several appointments with the timing individualised for each patient and family. Adult DSD services should have a gynaecologist, endocrinologist and psychologist as a minimum.

11.13.5   Support Groups

With the advent of the internet and social media, support groups have arisen [14]. Peer support is vitally important for those with rare conditions and can have a positive effect on well-being. This allows both individuals with DSD and families to connect and share experiences. It also has promoted activist groups, who have views on provision of medical care, such as childhood genital surgery. Whilst activist groups can raise the profile of rare conditions and provide a much-needed voice from the patient community, it also cannot be assumed this represents all those with DSDs. Care should be taken to canvass the views and thoughts of individual patients regarding all aspects of their care.

11.14   Conclusion

The clinical management for those with DSDs has come a long way in the last two decades. Nowadays individuals and families will have full explanation and knowledge of their condition, and thanks to genetic advances are highly likely to have an accurate diagnosis. However, with this comes more challenges. There is a lack of data for older women with DSDs especially regarding health concerns after the menopause. In addition, in an age of social media, girls and women need to decide how and when to discuss their diagnosis with partners or friends. Those with DSDs require lifelong care including psychological support in order to meet the challenges for the future.

Key Learning Points

- DSDs are rare conditions which require an expert multidisciplinary team to coordinate and offer care.
- Initial investigations include a karyotype, ultrasound scan and hormone tests, with subsequent genetic tests being likely to identify a diagnosis.
- Surgery for those with atypical genitalia is controversial, and current practice may change.
- Gonadectomies are offered following completion of puberty, unless a significant malignant risk exists.
- Psychological care is mandatory and is often the most pressing need.

References

1. Lee PA, Houk CP, Ahmed SF, Hughes IA. Consensus statement on management of intersex disorders. Chicago Pediatr. 2006;**118**(2):e488–500.

2. Ahmed SF, Achermann JC, Arlt W, Balen A, Conway G, Edwards Z, et al. Society for Endocrinology UK guidance on the initial evaluation of an infant or an adolescent with a suspected disorder of sex development (revised 2015). Clin Endocrinol (Oxf). 2016;**84**(5):771–88.

3. Cools M, Nordenström A, Robeva R, Hall J, Westerveld P, Flück C, et al. Caring for individuals with a difference of sex development (DSD): a consensus statement. Nat Rev Endocrinol. 2018;**14**(7):415–29.

4. Once a dark secret. BMJ. 1994;**308**:542.

5. Roll MF, Kneppo C, Roth H, Bettendorf M, Waag KL, Holland-Cunz S. Feminising genitoplasty: one-stage genital reconstruction in congenital adrenal hyperplasia: 30 years' experience. Eur J Pediatr Surg. 2006;**16**(5):329–33.

6. Crouch NS, Liao LM, Woodhouse CR, Conway GS, Creighton SM. Sexual function and genital sensitivity following feminizing genitoplasty for congenital adrenal hyperplasia. J Urol. 2008;**179**(2):634–8.

7. Minto CL, Liao KL, Conway GS, Creighton SM. Sexual function in women with complete androgen insensitivity syndrome. Fertil Steril. 2003;**80**(1):157–64.

8. Chaudhry S, Tadokoro-Cuccaro R, Hannema SE, Acerini CL, Hughes IA. Frequency of gonadal tumours in complete androgen insensitivity syndrome (CAIS): a retrospective case-series analysis. J Pediatr Urol. 2017;**13**(5):498.

9. Deans R, Creighton SM, Liao LM, Conway GS. Timing of gonadectomy in adult women with complete androgen insensitivity syndrome (CAIS): patient preferences and clinical evidence. Clin Endocrinol (Oxf). 2012;**76**(6):894–8.

10. Liao LM, Tacconelli E, Wood D, Conway G, Creighton SM. Adolescent girls with disorders of sex development: a needs analysis of transitional care. J Pediatr Urol. 2010;**6**(6):609–13.

11. Ismail-Pratt IS, Bikoo M, Liao LM, Conway GS, Creighton SM. Normalization of the vagina by dilator treatment alone in complete androgen insensitivity syndrome and Mayer–Rokitansky–Kuster–Hauser syndrome. Hum Reprod. 2007;**22**(7):2020–4.

12. Routh JC, Laufer MR, Cannon GM Jr, Diamond DA, Gargollo PC. Management strategies for Mayer–Rokitansky–Kuster–Hauser related vaginal agenesis: a cost-effectiveness analysis. J Urol. 2010;**184**(5):2116–21.

13. Crouch NS, Creighton SM. Transition of care for adolescents with disorders of sex development. Nat Rev Endocrinol. 2014;**10**(7):436–42.

14. www.dsdfamilies.org/charity.

Premature Ovarian Insufficiency

Lina Michala

12.1 Introduction

Premature Ovarian Insufficiency (POI) is defined by follicular depletion that occurs under the age of 40 and is characterised by a gradual fall of hormone production by the ovary, leading to amenorrhoea and infertility. The hallmark for diagnosis is raised follicle-stimulating hormone (FSH) above 25 IU/L measured twice, at least 4 weeks apart.

Ovarian ageing normally leads to the menopause at an average of 51 years. The time of oocyte depletion is determined by the number of oocytes that has populated the ovary during embryonic life and the rate of atresia that starts prior to birth and continues until the menopause.

12.2 Clinical Presentation

POI occurs in about one in 100 women under the age of 40. It can, however, present at any age, albeit with a decreased incidence. Specifically, it is estimated that POI affects 1 in 1000 women under the age of 30 and about 1 in 10,000 women under the age of 20 years. It can therefore present in adolescence with pubertal delay, primary or secondary amenorrhoea or dysfunctional uterine bleeding (DUB) due to anovulatory cycles.

In adolescence these symptoms are often mistaken for physiological or idiopathic changes and the diagnosis may thus be delayed or masked by the administration of hormonal contraceptive methods.

POI presents a spectrum of symptoms, with shorter follicular phases, anovulation and DUB often preceding the final stage of complete ovarian silence, which is characterised by amenorrhoea.

During early stages of failure, gonadotrophin, specifically follicle-stimulating hormone (FSH), is often within a normal range. When looking closely at laboratory results, however, this is usually secondary to the production of increased oestrogen due to the presence of a functional follicular cyst or a shorter follicular phase. Therefore, high levels of estradiol during the follicular phase may be an early indirect sign of ovarian dysfunction.

During early stages, ultrasonography may reveal a smaller ovarian volume and a reduced antral follicular count or follicular cysts, whereas at a final stage, ovaries are devoid of follicles and the endometrium is thin, as a result of low oestrogen levels.

Anti-Müllerian hormone (AMH) may be used when there is suspicion of an early-stage POI and gonadotrophin levels are inconclusive. However, normal values vary depending on the stage of pubertal development, and even with lower than expected levels, it is not possible to provide a safe prediction of the rate of ovarian decline [1].

12.3 Aetiology

POI may be congenital (chromosomal or genetic) or acquired (iatrogenic, infectious or autoimmune). In over 50% of cases, however, the aetiology will not be identified.

Certain known causes of POI are shown in Table 12.1.

- Turner syndrome is the commonest chromosomal disorder identified in women with POI, affecting one in 2000 births. Diagnosis is often made antenatally, in the newborn period or childhood as a result of investigations for increased nuchal thickness, congenital cardiac anomalies, limb lymphoedema or a short stature. However, diagnosis in approximately one-third of girls will be triggered through investigations for delayed puberty and/or primary amenorrhoea.

    Turner syndrome is characterised by streak ovaries, due to an increased rate of follicular atresia. Some girls, particularly those with a Turner mosaicism, may actually retain ovarian function and develop into puberty normally. The

Table 12.1 Indicative causes of POI

Chromosomal	Turner syndrome and mosaicisms	47XXX	46XY (Swyer syndrome)	
Genetic conditions	Fragile X syndrome	Galactosaemia, BPES (FOXL2)	FSH receptor mutation	NR5A1, STAG3, BMP15, ELF2B
Autoimmune	Steroid-producing cells	Myasthenia gravis	SLE	
Systemic infections	Mumps			
Iatrogenic causes	Radiation	Chemotherapy	Oophorectomy Surgery to the ovary	

majority, however, will eventually later develop POI and secondary amenorrhoea.

Girls diagnosed with TS should be under regular follow-up for acquired autoimmune, metabolic and cardiac conditions, as discussed in Chapter 10.

- Fragile X gene (FMR1) is located on the X chromosome and normally has under 45 CGG repeats at the N end of the allele. A full mutation is characterised by the presence of more than 200 repeats and leads to severe mental restriction, whereas in a premutation, repeats of 55–200 cause POI in approximately one-fourth of cases [2].

Fragile X premuations are more likely to be found in families where there is a strong history of POI or dementia.

- A multitude of genetic mutations have been implicated in POI. In certain cases, the causative mutation is already known when POI is identified. For example, **galactosaemia** [3] leads to POI in the majority of affected girls and is usually identified at birth. Syndromic features, such as those seen in **blepharophimosis syndrome** [4], are again indicative of specific gene mutations in women with POI. In other cases, gene mutations lead to gonadal dysgenesis, which usually presents with complete ovarian silence and first becomes evident with delayed puberty. Finally, certain other genetic conditions may be more common among certain populations, such as a mutation of the FSH receptor gene more commonly seen among Finnish women with POI, where follicular reserve is not affected but no oestradiol production is seen by the ovary due to **resistance to FSH** [5]. These women present with delayed puberty and despite raised FSH levels they will have normal ovaries on imaging and a normal AMH level.

- Adrenocortical antibodies lead to an autoimmune form of POI where there is lymphocytic infiltration of secondary follicles, leading to a selective destruction of theca cells. As granulosa cells remain unaffected, there is a paradoxically normal AMH, despite elevated FSH levels. On ultrasound the ovary may appear normal, as primary follicles remain intact.

Women with autoimmune POI are at risk of developing adrenocortical insufficiency, and should be thus referred to an endocrinologist to rule out Addison's disease [6].

- Increasingly a number of young women will present into adolescence with ovarian insufficiency due to chemotherapy or radiation received in childhood for cancer treatment. Iatrogenic causes of POI are on the increase due to the increased survival rate of childhood cancer [7].

- Mumps virus causes oophoritis, leading to transient ovarian failure. It is possible that other viral illnesses can also lead to POI, but it is often difficult to link the disease to POI as it may have been subclinical or presented long before POI is identified.

- It is possible that many idiopathic cases of POI are due to either unknown genetic conditions or prior viral illnesses.

12.4 Diagnostic Algorithm

POI should be investigated as a cause of delayed puberty, primary or secondary amenorrhoea or where dysfunctional uterine bleeding persists beyond 2–3 years after menarche or presents in a woman that previously had regular cycles.

Confirmatory diagnosis of POI is made when FSH levels are above 25 IU/L in two consecutive measurements more than 4 weeks apart.

When POI is identified, the following investigations should be performed:

- Karyotype
- Fragile X premutations
- Adrenocortical antibodies
- Thyroid antibodies

A diagnosis of Turner syndrome should lead to a series of baseline investigations to rule out congenital or acquired cardiovascular disease, along with regular investigations for the development of metabolic and autoimmune disease.

Prior to performing genetic testing for fragile X premutations there should be extensive counselling regarding the implications of the diagnosis. In particular, other family members may need to be tested, and if women are identified as carriers they would also be at risk of developing POI or of delivering a boy with a fragile X mutation and potentially severe learning difficulties.

Specific genetic investigations for POI other than fragile X premutations are currently not recommended except where there is a known condition within a family or syndromic features suggestive of a specific genetic mutation.

If adrenocortical antibodies are detected, then the woman should be referred to an endocrinologist as she is at risk of developing Addison's disease [8].

12.5 Management

15.5.1 Induction of Puberty

After puberty induction, which is achieved with the administration of gradually increasing doses of transdermal or oral oestrogen, and once a breakthrough vaginal bleeding occurs, the girl with POI will need hormonal replacement therapy (HRT) in the form of a combined preparation containing oestrogen and progesterone. (See also Chapters 3 and 10.)

12.5.2 Hormone Replacement Therapy, Dosage and Route of Administration

The transdermal route has the benefit of releasing oestrogen directly to the systemic rather than the portal circulation and provides steady levels of oestrogen in the bloodstream. Administration is either through patches or transdermal gel application and the dosage may range between 50 mcg and 200 mcg oestradiol per patch. Transdermal

HRT administration as opposed to oral has also the benefit of less adverse gastrointestinal effects, such as nausea and vomiting.

Nevertheless, many women find transdermal patches difficult to comply with, either because they are visible to others or because they cause local skin irritation.

When choosing the oral administration route, natural oestrogen-containing preparations are preferred over the combined oral contraceptive, which usually contains ethinylestradiol, as the latter interferes more with metabolism and clotting mechanisms. An alternative would be the usage of estradiol-containing oral contraceptive pills, which provide contraception and hormonal coverage.

The usual estradiol dose contained in generic oral HRT preparations is 2 mg. This dose has been designed mostly to cover the needs of older menopausal women, but this may not be sufficient to cater for the needs of a young woman with POI and the dose may need to be adjusted accordingly [9]. Measuring estradiol levels is not helpful in clinical practice, nor is monitoring FSH levels, which often do not normalise despite HRT treatment.

Progesterone is required to prevent endometrial hyperplasia and is always required as an adjuvant to oestrogen in women having a uterus. Progestogens can be administered orally, vaginally, intrauterine or transdermally. Natural progesterone can be used, although it is often associated with drowsiness and may not be well tolerated. Usually a synthetic progestogen such as norethisterone, dydrogesterone, medroxyprogesterone or drosperinone is preferred.

Progestogens are administered for 10–14 days a month, thus provoking a withdrawal bleed a few days after its cessation. If, however, the woman prefers not to have vaginal bleeding, she can take a continuous combined preparation that will provide a steady dose of progesterone throughout the cycle. Alternatively, systemic oestrogen can be combined with a levonorgestrel-releasing intrauterine system (LNG-IUS), which will also lead to bleed-free hormone replacement.

HRT reverses vasomotor symptoms and may improve well-being and vitality in oestrogen-deficient women. Titration of the dose is usually achieved through follow-up of symptoms, namely those suggesting persistent oestrogen deficiency, such as vasomotor symptoms, tiredness, sleep disturbances, and those suggesting increased dosage, such as headaches, nausea, breast tenderness. Withdrawal bleeding patterns should also be assessed, as excessive or protracted bleeding may be an indication to increase or change progestogen coverage to one that stabilises the endometrium better. However, progestogens such as norethisterone lead to stronger androgenic side effects, such as acne and hirsutism, which can be particularly bothersome.

Titration is also achieved through monitoring of bone density scans at regular intervals.

12.5.2.1 Monitoring and Duration of Treatment

Because of the long-term risks of osteoporosis [10] and cardiovascular disease [11] it is essential to promote a healthy lifestyle, emphasising a diet containing calcium-rich foods, smoking cessation and regular aerobic and weight-bearing exercising.

Bone mineral density should be measured at baseline and then at regular frequent intervals, every 2–3 years, to monitor bone mass accrual during adolescence and young adulthood. Women with POI are often deficient with regard to bone density, and this is particularly a problem for women diagnosed early on, or those that are smokers, lead a sedentary life, have a low body mass index (BMI) or have reduced levels of vitamin D or are deficient in calcium intake.

It is important to monitor for vitamin D deficiency as well as blood pressure during annual visits. Depending on body mass index (BMI) and family and personal medical history, serum lipids and blood sugar levels should also be checked at regular intervals.

Treatment with HRT is usually continued until the average age of menopause. At yearly consultation the preparation, dosage and route of administration should be re-evaluated.

12.6 Psychosexual Well-being

POI is a devastating diagnosis with multiple repercussions to general health and sexuality.

To a certain extent, these can be reversed through HRT, which will alleviate vasomotor symptoms and improve sleep disturbances and tiredness. Oestrogen replacement may also improve mild mood disorders related to POI as cerebral serotonin levels are restored [12]. Lifestyle interventions such as dietary changes, exercise and better sleep habits could improve well-being. Formal psychological counselling should be offered to help come to terms with the diagnosis and overcome difficulties associated with the condition.

In young girls and women who are sexually active, vaginal atrophy can lead to dyspareunia. Women with POI may be reluctant to come forward with sexual or urogenital concerns, therefore it is important to assess for these symptoms through direct questioning at annual consultations or during routine vaginal examinations. Systemic oestrogen improves symptomatology of vaginal dryness and atrophy but may need to be supplemented with local vaginal oestrogen. Nevertheless, women with POI will still have reduced sexual satisfaction even while taking HRT, thus indicating that psychological mechanisms may be involved.

Physiological transdermal testosterone supplementation has been used to improve well-being and sexuality. However, treatment remains controversial and results are inconclusive [13].

12.7 Fertility Preservation and Future Fertility Prospects

In certain cases of POI, the diagnosis may be made before follicular depletion, thus giving an opportunity for fertility preservation through oocyte vitrification or ovarian tissue cryopreservation. This is possible for girls that have either been identified following the diagnosis of a parent or sibling with a genetic condition that leads to POI, such as fragile X premutation, or that are known to have a condition leading to POI such as the rare case of Turner syndrome with retained ovarian function.

Fertility preservation is also now offered as a routine in all young girls and women who will undergo gonadotoxic treatment, usually as part of cancer treatment.

A proportion of women with POI may achieve a spontaneous pregnancy. This is estimated to occur in approximately 4%–5% of women. Women who have been recently diagnosed with POI, have visible follicles on ultrasound or at times have spontaneous menstruation are more likely to fall pregnant. It is therefore recommended that women with POI continue to use contraception if they do not wish to conceive. In order to avoid contraceptive failure, the combined contraceptive pill should be used with no breaks in women with POI, as ovulation may occur during the 7-day break. Alternatively, a LNG-IUS can be inserted and combined with oral or transdermal oestrogen. Similarly, it is important to clarify that oral and transdermal HRT does not provide contraception.

The mainstay for achieving a pregnancy in women with POI is through oocyte donation [14]. Careful assessment for comorbidities should, however, be offered. In particular, women with Turner syndrome or those that have received anthracyclins or have had thoracic irradiation as part of cancer treatment in the past, should have a thorough cardiovascular evaluation prior to considering pregnancy [14,15].

12.8 Conclusion

POI can have serious implications for health and quality of life of women, both in the short and long run. It is important to identify women early, to institute treatment and modify their lifestyle so as to alleviate vasomotor symptoms, maintain bone mass density, reduce cardiovascular risk and improve urogenital and sexual health and well-being.

Spontaneous ovulation may still occur occasionally in a small percentage of women. Still, fertility at present cannot be improved and pregnancy is usually achieved through oocyte donation. Important work is currently being undertaken in identifying those at risk of developing POI so as to offer fertility preservation.

Key Learning Points

- POI is diagnosed when FSH levels are raised above 25 IU/L on two occasions measured 4 weeks apart in women under the age of 40.
- POI may be iatrogenic, due to a karyotype aberration, a genetic mutation or a viral illness. However, the majority are of unknown aetiology.
- When POI is diagnosed, it is recommended to perform a karyotype, to do a fragile X mutation screening and to test for adrenocortical and thyroid antibodies.
- HRT reverses vasomotor symptoms and helps maintain and improve bone mineral density, as well as cardiovascular health.

References

1. Kelsey TW, Wright P, Nelson SM, Anderson RA, Wallace WH. A validated model of serum anti-Müllerian hormone from conception to menopause. PLoS One. 2011;6(7):e22024.

2. Raspa M, Wheeler AC, Riley C. Public health literature review of fragile X syndrome. Pediatrics. 2017;139 (Suppl 3):S153–71.

3. Fridovich-Keil JL, Gubbels CS, Spencer JB, Sanders RD, Land JA, Rubio-Gozalbo E. Ovarian function in girls and women with GALT-deficiency galactosemia. J Inherit Metab Dis. 2011;34(2): 357–66.

4. Nuovo S, Passeri M, Di Benedetto E, Calanchini M, Meldolesi I, Di Giacomo MC, et al. Characterization of endocrine features and genotype-phenotypes correlations in blepharophimosis-ptosis-epicanthus inversus syndrome type 1. J Endocrinol Invest. 2016;39 (2):227–33.

5. Tapanainen JS, Vaskivuo T, Aittomäki K, Huhtaniemi IT. Inactivating FSH receptor mutations and gonadal dysfunction. Mol Cell Endocrinol. 1998;145 (1–2):129–35.

6. Bakalov VK, Vanderhoof VH, Bondy CA, Nelson LM. Adrenal antibodies detect asymptomatic auto-immune adrenal insufficiency in young women with spontaneous premature ovarian failure. Hum Reprod. 2002;17 (8):2096–100.

7. SIGN. Long term follow up of survivors of childhood cancer. Edinburgh: SIGN; 2013.

8. ESHRE Guideline: Management of women with premature ovarian insufficiency. Guideline of the European Society of Human Reproduction and Embryology. Hum Reprod. 2016;31(5):926–37.

9. Crofton PM, Evans N, Bath LE, Warner P, Whitehead TJ, Critchley HO, et al. Physiological versus standard sex steroid replacement in young women with premature ovarian failure: effects on bone mass acquisition and turnover. Clin Endocrinol (Oxf). 2010;73 (6):707–14.

10. Popat VB, Calis KA, Vanderhoof VH, Cizza G, Reynolds JC, Sebring N, et al. Bone mineral density in estrogen-deficient young women. J Clin Endocrinol Metab. 2009;94(7):2277–83.

11. van der Schouw YT, van der Graaf Y, Steyerberg EW, Eijkemans JC, Banga JD. Age at menopause as a risk factor for cardiovascular mortality. Lancet. 1996;347 (9003):714–8.

12. Epperson CN, Amin Z, Ruparel K, Gur R, Loughead J. Interactive effects of estrogen and serotonin on brain activation during working memory and affective processing in menopausal women. Psychoneuroendocrinology. 2012;37(3):372–82.

13. Guerrieri GM, Martinez PE, Klug SP, Haq NA, Vanderhoof VH, Koziol DE, et al. Effects of physiologic testosterone therapy on quality of life, self-esteem, and mood in women with primary ovarian insufficiency. Menopause. 2014;21(9):952–61.

14. Hadnott TN, Gould HN, Gharib AM, Bondy CA. Outcomes of spontaneous and assisted pregnancies in Turner syndrome: the US National Institutes of Health experience. Fertil Steril. 2011;95(7):2251–6.

15. van Dalen EC, van der Pal HJ, van den Bos C, Kok WE, Caron HN, Kremer LC. Clinical heart failure during pregnancy and delivery in a cohort of female childhood cancer survivors treated with anthracyclines. Eur J Cancer. 2006;42(15):2549–53.

Chapter 13

Gynaecological Laparoscopy in Adolescents

Thomas R. Aust and Alfred Cutner

13.1 Introduction

Laparoscopic surgery is open surgery carried out through small incisions with enhanced magnification of the operative field. The advantages of a laparoscopic (or keyhole) approach to the abdomen and pelvis have been well documented and include: a significant reduction in postoperative pain, length of stay, recovery time and adhesion formation. In children or adolescents this will result in a faster return to school and normal activities. Laparoscopic incisions are much smaller than a transverse incision and indeed a midline laparotomy. This reduction in wound visibility is especially important in children and adolescents who otherwise may be asked by contemporaries or a new partner about the reasons behind the scar. This will be especially distressing while coming to terms with the psychological impact of the diagnosis of an XY karyotype or an absent uterus.

The enhanced visualisation of laparoscopic surgery is due to the greater magnification and ability to see deep into the pelvis compared to open surgery. This is especially important in cases of Müllerian anomalies or endometriosis when the anatomy is distorted and access to the operative site is difficult to achieve.

The advantages of laparoscopic surgery for both the patient and the surgeon would indicate that this approach should be the technique of choice when operating within the abdomen and pelvis in paediatric and adolescent gynaecology (PAG).

13.2 Planning, Theatre Set-up and Equipment

13.2.1 Who Should Perform These Operations, and in What Location?

The make-up of the team will depend on the age and maturity of the patient and the condition with which they present. For example a 16-year-old with an ovarian cyst can be managed in a similar manner to a young adult in terms of anaesthetic and operative techniques. Conversely, a 12-year-old with a complex Müllerian duct anomaly or a difference of sex development may require a paediatric anaesthetist, paediatric urologist, paediatric surgeon, clinical psychologist and a paediatric endocrinologist. In addition the hospital environment for surgical recovery is important and needs to take into account the age of the patient and the potential need for parental support. A room covered in cartoon characters with lights-off at 7:00 PM will put a young child at ease but would not be appropriate for a teenager. However, in most units adolescents are not treated on adult wards as this is not the correct environment.

It would be unusual for an individual to have all the correct knowledge and skills required and hence a team approach is likely to optimise outcome. Some of the laparoscopic surgery will be complex and it is unlikely that an expert PAG consultant who deals with all other aspects of patient management will have a sufficient laparoscopic workload to enable adequate skill acquisition. Likewise an expert laparoscopic surgeon who carries out a heavy surgical workload is unlikely to have sufficient knowledge surrounding all the other aspects of care. Thus a team approach of a PAG specialist (with the correct knowledge) operating with an adult laparoscopic specialist with the skills of dissection of the pouch of Douglas, uterovesical fold and pelvic sidewall and proficiency in laparoscopic suturing will optimise the surgical outcome. This approach is common in units offering complex surgery to this group of patients in the United Kingdom. We would encourage anyone endeavouring to perform complex laparoscopy in the PAG setting to foster this working relationship.

13.2.2 Planning Surgery

The preoperative assessment in making the diagnosis and determining the indications for surgery are dealt with in the relevant chapters in the book. This section will address the surgery.

The suitability for laparoscopic surgery needs to take into account the specifics of the surgery itself and also general considerations. Previous abdominal surgery and the size of the patient may determine the method for obtaining a pneumoperitoneum. Previous abdominal surgery increases the risks of adhesions and hence organ damage during primary port insertion.

The requirement to use a uterine manipulator should be discussed with the patient and her family during the preoperative period, especially with girls who have never been sexually active. This may have significant social and religious implications, as there is a risk that the hymen may tear.

In procedures where there is a Müllerian duct anomaly preoperative knowledge of the renal tract is essential as it is important to know whether there is an absent kidney or a duplex system. This information will be required during surgical dissection of the pelvic sidewall. In XY females, preoperative MRI will in most cases locate the site of the gonads and hence enable preoperative planning of the surgical approach and potential requirements of a paediatric urologist where groin dissection may be required.

13.2.3 Theatre Set-up

Surgery requires an effective team with each member having a specific role. The familiarity of the anaesthetic, scrub and circulating staff with each other, with their equipment and with the procedures being performed will have a direct effect on the smooth running of each case.

The theatre environment has to be fit for purpose. Advanced laparoscopic theatre set-ups may reduce stress in the operating theatre and minimise risks to staff and patients. The layout of equipment in the operating room has become more important as the technology has increased. When open surgery was the norm a single diathermy machine and a suction bottle were the only devices that needed to be near the operating table. With laparoscopic surgery requirements include newer energy machines such as ultracision and advanced bipolar, insufflator stacks, suction/irrigation set-ups and multiple

high-definition monitors and control screens. The layout needs to facilitate flow of equipment to the operating table without obscuring the surgeons' view of the monitors. Ideally cables running along the floor should be minimised as they represent a trip-hazard in the low-light conditions of a laparoscopic theatre. Having an integrated system that allows the surgeon to control gas-flow, light intensity and the recording of images rather than requesting circulating staff to do it saves time and improves efficiency.

State-of-the-art theatres result in a quietly flowing theatre where staff feel less stressed, which allows the team to concentrate on the operation itself. This results in a more efficient and relaxed surgical environment, which enables more complex surgery to be carried out in a safer manner.

13.2.4 Laparoscopic Techniques and Equipment

Most laparoscopic pelvic procedures are performed in the Lloyd-Davies position to enable access to the vagina if required. Prior to insufflation the bladder is emptied either by an in-out catheter for short procedures or an indwelling catheter for longer procedures or ones in which the bladder has to be filled to help identify it. At the end of the procedure this can be removed if the operation was only minor. Consideration should be given to leaving the catheter overnight as trying to catheterise a child who goes into urinary retention postoperatively can be traumatic. If the uterus is present and the operation involves inspection of the pouch of Douglas or uterine manipulation, then the uterus is instrumented.

There are three main methods used to obtain a pneumoperitoneum: insertion of a Veres needle at the umbilicus, open entry (Hasson) and subcostal approach (Palmer's entry). Many patients in this age group will be more susceptible to vascular injury from a standard umbilical Veres technique due to the short distance from the umbilicus to the major abdominal blood vessels. To minimise the risk of vascular injury a Hasson entry technique should be considered especially in thin patients.

Umbilical entry is not suitable, whether via a closed or open technique, where there is an increased risk of adhesions under the umbilicus. An alternative entry site should be used. A Veres needle or a direct optical entry at Palmers point (left upper quadrant 2 cm below the costal margin) provides a relatively safe entry into the abdomen, allowing the inside of the umbilicus to be inspected and a port placed if free of adhesions. Where a subcostal entry point is utilised there is an increased risk of damaging the stomach if it is distended. An oro-gastric tube should be placed at the start of the operation.

Instrumentation would largely reflect the same used in adult surgery. Minimising the number and size of the ports should be considered to enhance the cosmetic result. However, this should not be at the expense of safe, efficient surgery. For most operations we utilise an umbilical 5 or 10 mm port for the laparoscope and 2 lateral ports in line with the umbilicus and very lateral. This enables good triangulation during surgery. For complex cases we also insert a suprapubic 5 or 10 mm port to enable additional manipulation by the assistant. In cases where further retraction would be useful we insert needles and suspend structures with sutures to carry this out without the need for extra ports.

13.3 Laparoscopic Management of Endometriosis

Dysmenorrhoea is a common condition affecting 40%–50% of teenagers. Making a diagnosis is difficult as symptoms can vary and there are no non-invasive tools to detect mild and moderate disease (i.e. no ovarian endometrioma or rectal nodule) prior to laparoscopic identification.

Diagnosing endometriosis in the PAG population is difficult as their symptoms may be atypical and include non-cyclic pain, vague acute abdominal symptoms, gastrointestinal and genito-urinary symptoms. Sexually active teenagers may also report dyspareunia. Furthermore, there can be confusion and crossover with other causes of pelvic pain such as irritable bowel syndrome, constipation and bladder pain syndromes.

Studies suggest that 69%–73% of teenagers whose pain was resistant to medical management (such as NSAIDS or progestogen-only or combined contraceptive pills) were found to have endometriosis so it is reasonable to only laparoscope those who don't respond to medical treatment. Those that do respond may still have endometriosis (around 50%) so it is important that these patients bear that in mind. The levonorgestrel intrauterine system (LNG-IUS) is a less invasive option which can also be considered, although it often requires a general anaesthetic for insertion in teenagers, especially if they have never been sexually active.

13.3.1 Appearance and Severity of Endometriosis

Most adolescents who have endometriosis (>60%) will have early-stage disease confined to the pelvis but advanced endometriosis has been described. A major risk factor of disease severity is a Müllerian duct anomaly resulting in an outflow obstruction. The incidence of endometriosis in this group of adolescents with genital tract anomalies varies between 6% and 40%. Surgical treatment of the outflow obstruction will often result in improvement or even spontaneous resolution so many surgeons do not treat the endometriosis at the initial operation. The risk of severe disease also appears to increase with advancing age and early menarche and this goes along with the thinking that endometriosis is a progressive disease that gets worse with increasing number of menstrual cycles.

It should be noted, however, that adolescents with endometriosis often have subtle atypical lesions that are clear, white or red, and not the powder-burn lesions commonly seen in adults. Familiarity with atypical lesions is important at the time of laparoscopy in making the correct diagnosis.

The goal of laparoscopic surgery is to make a diagnosis and to treat the disease conservatively in the hope of reducing pain whilst preserving fertility. Treatment with either resection or ablation of endometriotic lesions and postoperative medical therapy has been shown to result in clinical improvement in symptoms. However, in adults the evidence suggests that excision may be better than ablation when treating endometriosis and that is the approach taken by the authors. An early diagnosis is believed by many authors to be an opportunity to intervene in the progressive nature of the disease. Unfortunately, the recurrence of pain and/or disease is a significant problem and appears to occur regardless of postoperative adjuvant therapy. It is not surprising that the need for a second operation to treat recurrent symptoms has been reported to be as high as 34% 5 years postoperatively in adolescent patients.

13.4 Laparoscopic Management of Benign Ovarian Masses

13.4.1 General Considerations

The first consideration when deciding on surgical treatment of a presumed benign ovarian mass in children is preservation of ovarian function. An ovarian cystectomy is always preferred over an oophorectomy as many follicles are left behind after cystectomy and can serve as oocytes for reproduction in the future.

Among adolescents, the most common benign ovarian masses are functional cysts and benign neoplasms. There is a bimodal distribution of functional cysts, peaking during the fetal/neonatal and perimenarchal ages. As these cysts are usually benign and resolve spontaneously, every effort should be made to manage these cysts expectantly with serial ultrasound prior to considering surgery.

Paratubal and paraovarian cysts may mimic simple ovarian cysts in both presentation and imaging. Surgical management is usually suggested for any adnexal cyst greater than 5 cm that fails to regress. Surgical intervention will prevent potential torsion as well as provide a histological diagnosis. Fortunately, the majority of ovarian cysts can be managed by laparoscopy.

Neoplastic ovarian masses in the paediatric and adolescent population include tumours of germ cell, epithelial, sex cord stromal and metastatic from other primary sites. Germ cell tumours are the most common histological subtype in adolescents. Because non-epithelial masses predominate in the adolescent, the following discussion will focus on the most common benign germ cell tumour, the mature cystic teratoma.

13.4.2 Dermoid Cysts

Mature cystic teratomas, or dermoid cysts, arise from ectodermal, mesodermal and endodermal tissue and are the most common benign ovarian tumour found in children and adolescents. They frequently contain squamous epithelium containing sebaceous glands, sweat glands and hair follicles. When opened they release hair and sebaceous material, hence the name dermoid cyst. The majority of surgeons agree that symptomatic, large and atypical dermoids require surgical removal. In asymptomatic patients, the age of the patient, future fertility and cyst size are considered when deciding if surgery is indicated.

The increased risk of intraoperative cyst rupture remains the main disadvantage for considering a laparoscopic approach. Intraoperative rupture may result in a theoretical risk of chemical peritonitis, spillage of malignant cells into the peritoneal cavity, and/or adhesion formation. Fortunately, many studies have failed to demonstrate any complications of chemical peritonitis following spillage of dermoid

contents, supporting a minimally invasive approach. Laparoscopic cystectomy is the preferred method of treating dermoid cysts, with the aim of preserving as much ovarian tissue as possible. Bilateral dermoids occur in 10%–15% of cases, therefore the contralateral ovary should always be assessed at the time of surgery.

13.4.3 Adnexal Torsion

If torsion is suspected, prompt diagnosis and intervention is necessary to avoid long-term damage to the ovary and prevent oophorectomy. In cases of suspected ovarian torsion, detorsion with or without cystectomy has become the recommended surgical practice, even with a necrotic appearance of the ovary, as venous congestion can give a blue/black appearance when the ovary is still viable. Despite this recommendation, oophorectomy is still performed frequently at the time of ovarian torsion (30%–86%).

Historically, it was recommended to remove the adnexa due to a theoretical risk that untwisting the ovarian pedicle would result in a thromboembolic event. Large retrospective series of detorsion have failed to demonstrate any patients with a thromboembolic event, further supporting a conservative surgical approach.

The presence of a large ovarian mass (>8 cm) or suspected malignancy may preclude a laparoscopic approach but, fortunately, malignant lesions are particularly uncommon (<3%) in both the paediatric and adult populations.

Multiple studies have reported ovarian salvage following detorsion of the blue/black ovary. Ovarian function has been documented at the time of follow-up ultrasound, following additional surgery, or following successful IVF.

Risk of repeat torsion or torsion of the other ovary is a major concern. Prophylactic oophoropexy should be discussed at the time of surgery. The long-term effects of oophoropexy on future fertility are uncertain. Most surgeons consider performing this procedure when the ovarian ligament is congenitally long, in cases of repeat torsion, or when no obvious cause for the torsion is found. If an oophoropexy is carried out, the ovary is usually fixed to the pelvic sidewall, back of the uterus, or the ipsilateral uterosacral ligament with either absorbable or non-absorbable suture. Alternatively, the utero-ovarian ligament can be shortened (Figure 13.1).

13.5 Gonadectomy, Vaginoplasty and Complex Müllerian Duct Anomalies

13.5.1 Gonadectomy

The investigations and timing of gonadectomy in girls with a 46XY disorder of sex development has been discussed elsewhere. In most situations, the surgery will be carried out in late adolescence, once puberty is complete (Figure 13.2). There are two important factors that need to be considered when undertaking the surgery: The first is to ensure complete excision of the gonads and the second is their preoperative localisation.

Due to the potential malignant transformation of any residual tissue it is essential to ensure complete excision. Thus it is recommended to remove the fallopian tubes and to take both vascular pedicles a reasonable distance away from the gonadal tissue.

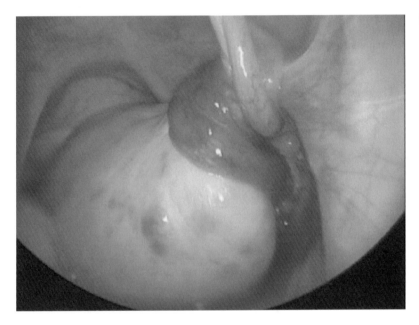

Figure 13.1 Torted right ovary.

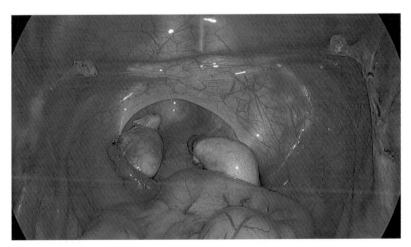

Figure 13.2 Gonadectomy in a girl with 46XY complete androgen insensitivity syndrome. Note the absent Müllerian structures.

The gonad can lie in any position along the normal path of descent of a testis in the male. In addition it may be streak in nature making identification difficult. Where the gonad lies in the inguinal canal, a urologist will remove it through a groin incision. However, at times, with massage of the groin and traction on the pedicle from the pelvic aspect, the gonad can be drawn back into the abdomen and removed laparoscopically. Conversely the gonad may lie higher up than expected and indeed outside the pelvis. Thus the operation may be straightforward at times but on other occasions require dissection around the ureter or sidewall vessels.

A method to occlude the pedicle and then divide it is required. Technologies such as re-usable bipolar and scissors may be employed but more advanced energy sources that utilise ultrasonic energy make the surgery easier and more efficient. Where the pedicle is close to the ureter the sidewall should be opened and formal separation carried out to prevent ureteric injury due to heat spread. At the end of the procedure it is preferable to remove the gonads separately, as if the histology were to demonstrate malignant transformation it is important to identify from which gonad it arose. Depending on whether or not a cyst was present on the gonad and hence the size, it may or may not be necessary to employ an extraction bag to remove the gonads from the abdomen.

13.5.2 Laparoscopic Creation of a Neovagina

The majority of women with a short blind-ending vagina (from conditions such as Mayer–Rokitansky–Küster–Hauser syndrome and complete androgen insensitivity syndrome) are able to use dilators with good effect. However, 15% will not get a satisfactory result or struggle with dilators especially if the perineum is flat with no vaginal dimple. These women can be offered a surgical procedure to create a functioning vagina. Most techniques were originally developed using laparotomy but are now performed laparoscopically.

13.5.2.1 Laparoscopic Vecchietti

The space between the bladder and rectum is opened so that a needle loaded with a suture can be passed into the pelvis from the vaginal dimple. A small acrylic olive is threaded and positioned in the vaginal dimple. The two ends of the thread are pulled from the vaginal dimple through the anterior abdominal wall and into a traction device. A cystoscopy is performed to exclude a bladder perforation during needle passing. The original description of this procedure suggests that the threads should be passed in a retroperitoneal fashion, but in our experience a trans-peritoneal path causes no problems. The device holds the threads under tension and, by turning a screw, shortens the threads evenly by 1 cm/d. This causes the olive to be pulled upwards, creating an elongation of the vagina over a week; at which point the traction device and beads are removed. The patient has a Foley catheter until the traction device is removed. Postoperative dilation and/or intercourse are required to maintain vaginal length.

13.5.2.2 Laparoscopic Davydov

In women who have no vaginal dimple or whose external genitalia are very scarred (e.g. from perineal surgery around birth/infancy) a Davydov procedure can be performed. The space between the rectum and bladder is developed both from the perineum below and laparoscopically from above. The edges of the pelvic peritoneum are 'pulled down' and attached to the dissected perineal skin with interrupted sutures to form a vagina lined with peritoneum. The open apex of the vagina is closed with an absorbable purse-string suture placed 11–13 cm from the opening of the neovagina. The peritoneum within the neovagina is replaced by squamous vaginal epithelium over the subsequent few months. This procedure would be difficult in patients who have undergone extensive abdominal surgery, as the peritoneum may not be sufficiently pliable to pull it down to the perineum.

13.5.2.3 Laparoscopic Intestinal Vaginoplasty

In patients who have previously had major abdominal surgery (such as bladder reconstruction for cloacal anomalies) intestinal vaginoplasty can be offered via a laparoscopic-assisted approach. A segment of bowel (usually sigmoid colon) is resected keeping its mesentery intact with one end of the bowel brought down to the perineum and sutured into place. Mucus production from the intestine can help with lubrication during intercourse, but some women have to douche to get rid of excessive secretions.

13.5.2.4 Deciding Which Procedure to Use

Choosing which form of neovagina to offer depends on many factors and should only be considered if the woman is sufficiently motivated and psychologically ready. It makes sense to offer the least invasive procedure initially so dilators should be offered before any surgical procedure is discussed. The choice of laparoscopic procedure will depend on history of previous surgery and the algorithm used by University College London Hospital aids the decision-making process (Figure 13.3).

Now that uterine transplantation has become a potential reality for women with uterine agenesis, the suitability of any neovagina to be connected to the transplanted cervix may need to be borne in mind in future. Ideally, a simple neovagina made of skin, which doesn't have the rectum or bladder in close approximation to the vault would probably be the easiest to attach to a transplanted uterus.

Neovaginas formed using dilation or laparoscopically will lack apical support and so are at risk of prolapse. A vault prolapse occurring in this situation would normally be repaired using the same technique as in a sacrocolpopexy for post-hysterectomy vault prolapse. The risk of prolapse should be part of the counselling process before surgery.

13.5.3 Müllerian Duct Anomalies

Abnormal development of the Müllerian structures can lead to various structural anomalies, many of which need no treatment particularly if asymptomatic. Anomalies that cause obstruction of menstrual flow such as a non-communicating uterine horn,

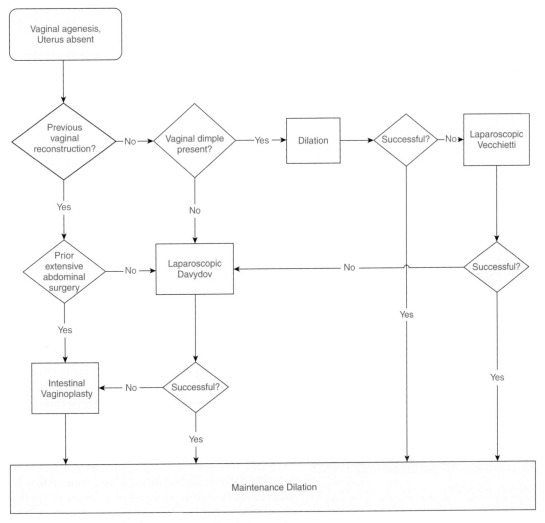

Figure 13.3 UCLH guide for the management of vaginal agenesis.

cervical agenesis or transverse vaginal septa can present with severe menstrual pain, or cyclical pain and primary amenorrhea if there is no normally communicating horn present. The age of onset of pain and its severity may vary considerably. This probably depends on the distensibility of the space into which the blood flows, the amount of retrograde flow of blood from the horn into the peritoneal cavity and the patient's perception of what is 'normal' period pain. Occasionally presentation is secondary to acute retention of urine from pressure from the haematocolpos.

13.5.3.1 Obstructed Uterine Horn

Treatment is by surgical excision of the horn. This is to improve pain and to remove the risk of cornual (i.e. uterine horn) ectopic pregnancy. The attached fallopian tube should also be removed to avoid the risk of an ectopic pregnancy from trans-peritoneal migration of sperm from the contralateral side. If the obstructed horn lies away from the functioning uterus then the procedure is simple. However, if the horn is adjacent to the functioning uterus and covered by myometrium then removal of the horn (and all of its endometrium and any rudimentary cervix) can be more challenging. The uterus can be extracted using mechanical morcellation. Preoperative imaging should ensure that the surgeon knows what to expect in terms of horn position and also the number of ureters and their location. See Figure 13.4.

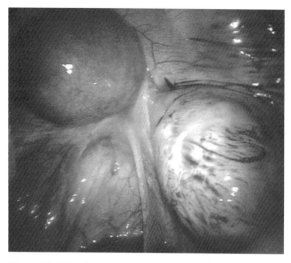

Figure 13.4 An obstructed right uterine horn. The distension from accumulated menstrual blood is evident when compared with the non-obstructed left side.

Women left with a unicornuate uterus should be warned that they are at increased risk of late miscarriage, preterm labour and malpresentation/position in any subsequent pregnancy.

13.5.3.2 Cervical Agenesis

Historically this condition was treated by hysterectomy to solve the pain of obstructed menstruation. More recently fertility-sparing surgery to perform a utero-vaginal anastomosis has been performed via laparotomy and laparoscopically. The procedure involves a combined laparoscopic and perineal approach. From above, the bladder is reflected from the uterus and a sound is introduced via the fundus to identify the level of obstruction. The distal end of the obstruction is canalised from the perineum with a combination of sharp and blunt dissection. The fibromuscular tissue at the level of the obstruction is then resected and the distal uterus connected to the upper vagina in a combined laparoscopic and perineal approach. A Foley catheter is left (deflated) in the uterine cavity extending into the vagina to prevent stenosis of the new canal, which is removed under anaesthetic about 1 month later.

13.5.3.3 Transverse Vaginal Septa

In cases where the obstructing septum is low in the vagina excision is performed via a vaginal approach. In cases of high vaginal septum a combined abdomino-perineal approach must be utilised. An algorithm has been published enabling a decision tree for the correct surgical approach (Figure 13.5).

In cases where the vagina and uterus are very distended, a Palmer's point entry is advisable. The utero-vesical peritoneum is opened and the bladder reflected down. The anterior aspect of the distended obstructed vagina is opened transversely and the haematocolpos drained. The transverse vaginal septum can then be excised and the incision enlarged from below using Hegar dilators. A device such as a McCartney tube can then be used to maintain the pneumoperitoneum. The proximal and distal vaginas can then be anastomosed using interrupted absorbable sutures. This can either be performed vaginally or laparoscopically depending on the vaginal access.

The anterior vaginal defect is then sutured laparoscopically. A vaginal pack and catheter are left in situ overnight.

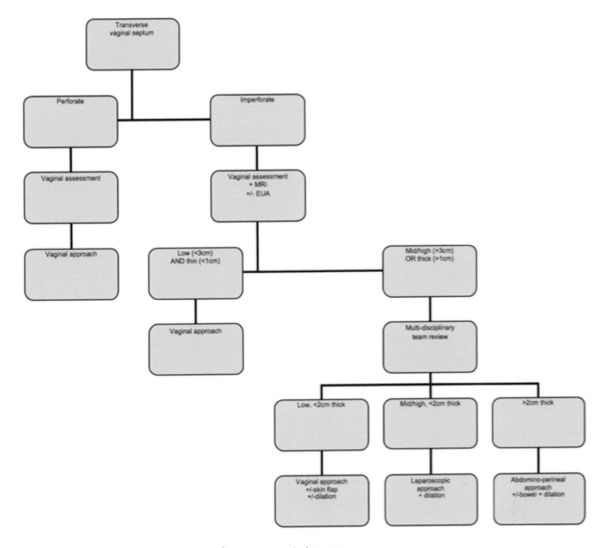

Figure 13.5 UCLH guide to the management of a transverse vaginal septum.

Key Learning Points

- Laparoscopic surgery should be the approach for most abdominal gynaecological procedures in the adolescent.
- A diagnostic (and potentially therapeutic) laparoscopy should be considered for those adolescents whose symptoms may suggest endometriosis and who do not respond to medical management.
- In cases of suspected adnexal torsion, prompt laparoscopy and detorsion should be performed and the ovary left in situ, as it will often remain viable even if it has a blue/black appearance.
- Creation of a neovagina can be performed through a minimally invasive approach if an attempt at dilation has failed. The method chosen depends on the underlying condition, previous surgery and the experience of the surgeons involved.
- Müllerian duct anomalies that cause obstruction of menstrual flow can cause pain that may require surgical intervention. These should be managed in a specialist centre.

References

1. Royal College of Obstetricians and Gynaecologists. Preventing entry-related gynaecological laparoscopic injuries. Green-Top Guideline 49. www.rcog.org.uk/en/guidelines-research-services/guidelines/gtg49/.

2. Duffy JMN, Arambage K, Correa FJS, Olive D, Farquhar C, Garry R, et al. Laparoscopic surgery for endometriosis. Cochrane Database Syst Rev. 2014;4:CD011031.

3. Sarıdoğan E. Adolescent endometriosis. Eur J Obstet Gynecol Reprod Biol. 2017;209:46–9.

4. Ismail I, Cutner A, Creighton S. Laparoscopic vaginoplasty: alternative techniques in vaginal reconstruction. BJOG. 2006;113:340–3.

5. Brännström M, Johannesson L, Bokström H, Kvarnström N, Mölne J, Dahm-Kähler P, et al. Livebirth after uterus transplantation. Lancet. 2015;385(9968):607–16.

6. Vallerie AM, Breech LL. Update in Müllerian anomalies: diagnosis, management, and outcomes. Curr Opin Obstet Gynecol. 2010;22(5):381–7.

7. Creighton SM, Davies MC, Cutner A. Laparoscopic management of cervical agenesis. Fertil Steril. 2006;85(5):1510.

14

Psychology in Paediatric and Adolescent Gynaecology

Julie Alderson and Samantha Cole

Clients and the general public are negatively affected by the continued and continuous medicalisation of the natural and normal responses to their experiences; responses which undoubtedly have distressing consequences which demand helping responses, but do not reflect illness so much as normal individual variation. [1, p. 2]

14.1 Introduction

Many young people seen in paediatric and adolescent gynaecology (PAG) clinics will be distressed and will be accompanied by distressed parents, carers or partners. Good multi-professional care can understand these natural and normal emotional and psychological responses. Aspects of physical development are increasingly characterised as natural variations rather than pathologies. Some previously routine PAG procedures, such as sex-affirming genital surgery, are now identified as socially motivated. All PAG practitioners need to develop a deeper understanding of those that are seeking their help to achieve optimal personal development.

14.2 A Psychologist on the Team

A PAG service should ideally have clinical or other practitioner psychologists as part of the multidisciplinary team (MDT). Others will have an associated clinical psychology service that will take patient referrals and report back. However, all gynaecologists working in PAG services or being referred young patients will need to incorporate an understanding of the psychological impact of young people's fears about their bodies in the presence or absence of any gynaecological condition. This chapter explains specialist integrated psychological care in PAG, but its other function is to develop the depth and breadth of the gynaecologist's psychologically informed thinking about patient care. We give advice on communicating with young people and families and signpost to useful resources.

There are different types of practitioner psychologist working within health care; for example, counselling psychologists and neuropsychologists. They have differ-

ent training and consequently their knowledge and skills vary. We will be focussing on clinical psychologists who complete a 6- to 9-year training involving doctoral research, are competent in a range of psychological therapies with different client or patient groups and have extensive assessment and formulation skills. Formulation uses psychological theory and evidence to understand thoughts, feelings and behaviours, how distress arises and is sustained, and to plan for change. It provides an individual, patient-specific picture of what is 'going on', why, and what might make a difference. Sharing and developing a formulation with a patient and a team can be a powerful psychological intervention; it opens doors to change, adaptation and acceptance, and helps the patient to adjust and recover with the wider medical team's understanding. Formulation shifts the patient from the passive position of having received a diagnosis and awaiting treatment or problem amelioration. This shared understanding approach can be used to meaningfully intervene with patients, their families and teams and can be applied throughout PAG and other physical health settings.

14.3 The Integrated Service Model of Psychological Care

Specialist psychology in physical health focusses the team on the mind – body interplay underpinning the patient's overall well-being. The psychologist's focus will be on helping the PAG team to understand the young person and their needs, including family and wider context issues. However, team function is not just a matter of linking up different experts to work together.

Box 14.1 The Psychologist as a Team Member

Psychologists can improve team processes and functioning by
- Facilitating team discussion of contentious issues
- Implementing patient experience improvements and coordinating interface with patient information, support and advocacy groups
- Co-working with other members of the team or providing uni-professional assessments or interventions
- Providing focussed individual or family therapeutic psychological work to allow patients to access routine aspects of care and
- Contributing to staff well-being activities

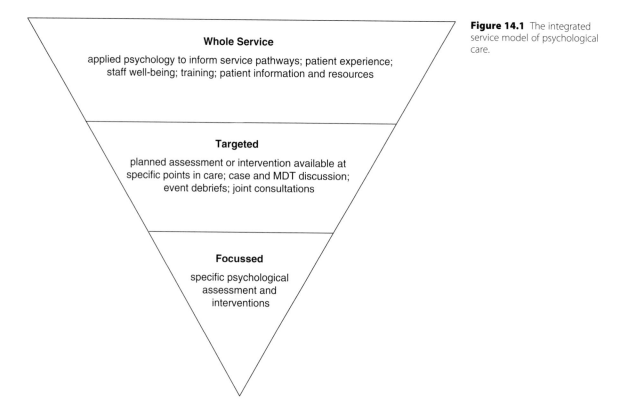

Whole Service

applied psychology to inform service pathways; patient experience; staff well-being; training; patient information and resources

Targeted

planned assessment or intervention available at specific points in care; case and MDT discussion; event debriefs; joint consultations

Focussed

specific psychological assessment and interventions

Figure 14.1 The integrated service model of psychological care.

Teams need to invest in the development of shared goals, agreed processes and ways to manage the intellectual- and emotional-relational processes involved in delivering meaningful psychological care [2,3].

The integrated psychology service model places multi-professional psychological care throughout the patient journey. The psychologist's focus will be on promoting patients' own understandings of their bodies and the team's understanding of each patient. By understanding the interplay between psychological and physical health, you can work together to prevent long-term problems and to promote good adaptation and a recovery-response to illness, injury or developmental variations. See Figure 14.1.

14.4 Whole-Service Psychological Care

The PAG psychologist can steer the psychological impact of the service for all patients, using screening tools, patient information and resources, and patient-reported experience or outcome measures (PROMs and PREMs). They can provide individual or group clinical supervision for nurses, service-wide teaching and facilitate challenging case discussions. They will bring psychological thinking to everyone's practice, advising on the impact of language or processes and liaising with peer support organisations to foster collaboration and promote self-management. Incorporating psychological aspects within research adds great value. Also, the impact of a specialist who can focus the service on promoting staff well-being easily translates to tangible patient benefit.

14.5 Staff Well-being

Box 14.2 The Impact of Compassion

Many studies demonstrate that even when doing so might represent an 'extra task', the time required to show meaningful compassion to patients is, on average, less than a minute. The fastest demonstrations of compassion tend to be those that are the most genuine. This genuine expression of compassion is associated with a measurable cumulative reduction in patient anxiety [8].

We know that when we fail to prioritise staff well-being we compromise effective care. Burnt-out staff risk providing depersonalised care [4] that is associated with lower-quality outcomes and increased risk of harm to patients from errors [5]. Organisational cultures that primarily focus on efficiency can engender a sense of threat in staff that can limit compassion by lowering clinicians' sensitivity to patient suffering and their motivation to address the suffering that they do become aware of [6]. Low compassion is associated with higher utilisation of resources and health care costs both because lower-quality care tends to be more expensive in the longer term and because clinicians that do not establish an understanding of patients' lived experience may be more reliant on avoidable testing and onwards referrals. Conversely, there is increasing evidence that teams with a culture of compassion are more effective. If patients feel cared for, their health outcomes are better [7]. Psychologists can play a major role in supporting staff to foster a culture of compassion and to become adept at practices and conversations that enact it.

14.6 Targeted Psychological Care

Within an MDT, a clinical psychologist can plan points along a care pathway where standard episodes of psychological care can be offered. These could be for every patient on a specific treatment path. For example, upon diagnosis of primary ovarian insufficiency (POI), patients could be given the opportunity to meet with the psychologist or a psychologically trained and supervised specialist nurse. This would have the specific aim of helping the young woman adapt, prepare for and get used to the lifelong consequences of the diagnosis and the possible personal responses, including a form of grief that can accompany an awareness of lost opportunities compared to previous expectations. Simultaneously, the patient's parents/carers might welcome advice on how best to support the young person, manage their own loss, and be signposted to support and self-management organisations. The PAG team psychologist could develop the offer of support, including co-designing information materials if none exist, providing clinical supervision for nurses, designing and evaluating pathways such as vaginal dilatation, developing and utilising specialist nurses' skills and coordinating the outcomes evaluation. Facilitating and evidencing routine patient involvement in decision-making is another aspect of targeted psychology provision. Involvement in decision-making places a person as an active contributor to their care. Being sure that the treatment is wanted by the patient, based on their understanding of the range of possible outcomes, including knowing how to help reach the best point using self-care is a great goal. Such patient and health professional concordance is more likely when patients and their parents are given flexibility and choice in shared decision-making [9,10].

In a well-developed PAG service, the psychologist would provide training and clinical supervision to the gynaecology specialist nurse who could then deliver psychologically informed care, only referring to the psychologist if they assess the need for focussed specialist psychological therapy. This type of proactive multi-professional care provides a compassionate, high-quality, whole-person service response to a life-altering diagnosis.

Box 14.3 Benefits of Targeted Psychological Care: Standard Pathway Provision

- Compassionate, whole-person service response to a life-altering diagnosis
- Patients who are fully supported to understand their bodies
- Patients who are aware of the support available via third-sector agencies
- Patients who are prepared for, and understand, their own psychological reactions
- A good level of concordance between patients and the team regarding the treatment plan
- Less likelihood of extended gynaecology follow-up due to high levels of distress involving information seeking

---

Box 14.4 Normative Pressure and Non-normative Care

PAG teams need to be responsive to the needs of non-binary people. For example, trans-men and trans-women may have health concerns pertaining to their vagina, neovagina, endocrinology or psychosexual health. It is common for socially transitioning people to consult PAG services whilst awaiting specialist gender identity services.

Irreversible surgical or medical interventions with young people that seek to achieve psychological goals should be made with extreme caution and in concert with robust psychological care due to the prevalence of gender fluidity across the lifespan.

14.7 Focussed Psychological Care

Some patients have specific psychological vulnerabilities that mean that the PAG diagnosis, treatment or even assessment and tests may trigger a more profound distress. A response to managing a long-term condition or a new diagnosis that shocks, might interrupt a patient's usual functioning. Some patients with no medical condition may present with a dissatisfaction with the normal development of their vulva. Others may experience a complicated grief reaction towards a diagnosis involving infertility, a shame reaction to learning about having internal testes, XY karyotype or in relation to managing vulval dermatitis. Some patients will be disappointed if you conclude that their concern, such as distress about the size or shape of labia, does not require physical treatment. In these situations a period of focussed psychological therapy can achieve greater psychological flexibility, enabling them to move to a stage where the targeted and service-wide psychological care is adequate or they can be discharged from the service.

In each of these situations, halting PAG care while sending the patient to generalist Child and Adolescent Mental Health Services (CAMHS) or Improving Access to Psychological Therapies (IAPT) services would be a disservice. Specialist psychological assessment and intervention that can work closely with nursing and gynaecology colleagues can provide knowledgeable, timely care that is acceptable to the patient, as part of her established care pathway. A clinical psychologist with specialist PAG knowledge who is part of the PAG team can advise you on how best to support the patient in line with the psychological work undertaken and can support you and the rest of the team to meet individual patient needs in the interest of optimal PAG outcomes. A clinical psychologist has skills in a range of therapies and interventions to draw on with patients, depending upon specific need and individual assessment. They can also swiftly assess risk of harm including suicidality or can help you sign-

---

Box 14.5 PAG Presentations That May Warrant Psychological Therapy

- A young woman with 21 hydroxyase deficiency congenital adrenal hyperplasia might have a period of difficulty adhering to her steroid regimen.
- A girl with Turner's mosaic might struggle to get used to wearing HRT patches or might have specific and distressing body image concerns.
- After experiencing childhood sexual assault, a woman with Mayer–Rokitansky–Küster–Hauser syndrome might agree to embark on a vaginal dilatation programme but experience flashbacks and distress when she holds the dilator towards her vulva.
- A young person may make persistent requests for surgical removal or reduction of their labia.

post to rapid response services if needed. They can also liaise with mental health service providers if a patient has ongoing mental health needs that do not directly pertain to their PAG condition. Occasionally, this will involve working with, or referring to, psychiatry colleagues while providing guidance on managing mental health comorbidities alongside gynaecological care.

14.8 Transition from Paediatric to PAG Care

One clear distinction within the PAG patient group will be on one hand those referred after long-term management by paediatric endocrinology or urology, and on the other, those coming to the PAG service to learn for the first time about aspects of their body and health. The former will include patients with a sex development diagnosis, some with unexpected genital difference at birth. Ideally, paediatric referral will involve extended pieces of co-management and service transition. The psychological and organisational complexity of the change in primary consultant and multi-professional team is largely hidden from families. The patient or family may expect the final 'handover' of care to instantly update PAG clinicians with all clinical details known to paediatricians. These expectations may increase the risk of patient disappointment or dissatisfaction and, therefore, intensifies the need for successful rapport building.

The transition period of overlap and joint working with a paediatric service provides impetus for a review and revision of physical and psychological care. The process presents an opportunity to take a history from the young person, sometimes with their parent/carer, that can help your patient learn all they can about their past, including how their parents handled their genital difference and any treatment decisions they contributed to. In separate PAG appointments, the team psychologist can use transition as a focus to help young patients take, and be given, increasing charge of their care. This family approach can help explore past parental/carer decisions about treatment and facilitate learning and understanding. For example, many young people and adults with variations in sex characteristics (sometimes called 'intersex' – a reclaimed term that many patients identify with – or medically categorised as DSD, an acronym for 'difference in sex development') report that they were not told about their bodies during childhood. In contemporary practice,

paediatric teams endeavour to be open with children whilst respecting parents'/carers' anxieties. While caring for children from birth to transition to PAG services, endocrinologists and sometimes urologists and psychologists will have negotiated with parents at each stage about who explains to a child about their body development. Ideally, children will have been supported to grow up (1) understanding their body, (2) knowing what physical treatments were discussed, (3) knowing what was decided upon and (4) what went ahead and (5) with what outcome. We have observed, however, that often parents require more psychological support than is generally available to be able to keep essential dialogue open with their children. A UK information and support charity dsdfamilies have published a guide for parents on 'Top Tips for Talking', available for download online [11]. The message here is that parents can build up from simple information based on an understanding of diversity, and as children grow older expand with information about the child's body and how it works. See Figure 14.2.

Where a young person has genital difference – whether or not parents agreed to genital surgery for their child in the past – it will be helpful to recapture family understanding of how they contributed to care decisions on behalf of their child. This support, offered at an anticipated point in the care pathway, is an example of 'targeted' care, available on specific pathways, as described above. This work, led by the PAG psychologist, can encourage the young person to establish a narrative about their body – past and future. With increasing autonomy for the young person, a full understanding of the rationale for any investigation or treatment might be expected by the PAG team but may be challenging for families who have been accustomed to parental decision-making. A team psychologist can help both parent and young person adjust. Ideally, parents will fully support their child to extend their knowledge and develop their autonomy. Since many parents experienced trauma during the neonatal period [12], memories are often triggered and fearful responses might result in tension during consultations.

14.9 Understanding the Silent and 'Un-knowing' or Distressed Patient

The Power, Threat, Meaning Framework (PTMF) is helpful for understanding the psychological responses

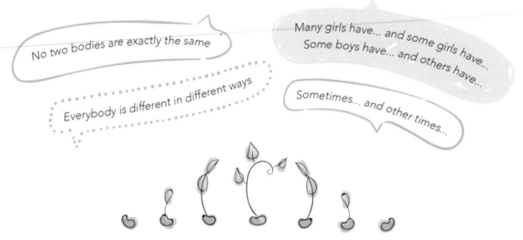

Figure 14.2 A model of sex differentiation from *The Story of Sex Development*. Reproduced with permission from dsdfamilies and Emily Tulloh, illustrator.

of patients or parents who may seem withdrawn, challenging or have difficult-to-understand behaviour [13]. The model recognises that people who have been subject to the power of others may struggle in similar threatening situations. The meaning of their distress, or the way they have learned to respond to threat, may be hidden to the people around them, or to themselves. The framework incorporates how messages from wider society can increase an individual's feelings of shame, self-blame, isolation, fear and guilt. For example, a parent who was traumatised by the reactions and language of health care professionals during their child's neonatal period, the extended period of time without information in response to their child's genital development, or the message to keep their child's genital development or chromosome pattern secret may experience refreshed trauma upon referral/transition to a PAG service. This may result in a high level of concern, mistrust and questioning.

A young woman learning for the first time that she has XY chromosomes and internal testes may be similarly traumatised by modes of information-giving without support or time to understand, counter her fears and adjust. It is common for young people to withdraw from services after diagnosis and engage in risky behaviours. Before looking at patient or parent reactions or communication style and hypothesising about or labelling their behaviour in mental health terms, think with compassion 'what happened and how have we responded'?

Consultations with a new patient at the time of a lifespan diagnosis can be very tense. Sometimes an explanation will confirm a family's fear, worry or concern and will culminate in shock or disbelief, with added uncertainties and unforeseen challenges. Fear can silence people and make them seem poorly informed. Even after reading about symptoms or speaking to their paediatric team and parents, rather than risk answering incorrectly, patients often respond cautiously. This approach may illicit from the doctor a re-telling or additional information. It is more likely that, when very uncomfortable or unsure, a young person will hesitate for an extended period or respond by saying very little.

Box 14.6 Don't Reach for a 'Mental Health' Label: Think 'Distress'

It is . . . not just psychiatric diagnosis and medicalisation as such, which needs to be fundamentally re-thought. . . . Modified versions such as the 'vulnerability-stress' or 'biopsychosocial' models still position social and relational factors as secondary to underlying biological causal malfunctions, and thus do not fully theorise distress as a *meaningful, functional and understandable response to life circumstances*. [13, p. 6, our italics]

Compassionate care based on empathy, kindness and a willingness to act may leave a health care professional open to one's own feelings of discomfort. Accepting that this is part of a commitment to thorough communication forms a foundation value for many in PAG services.

Young people who were diagnosed neonatally or in childhood with a rare diagnosis affecting sex development will have attended multiple clinic appointments along with their parents. Lifespan implications of the specific condition will have been discussed and interventions debated, planned and carried out with the child's knowledge; for example, the use of growth hormone. However, a history of paediatric care can still leave the patient and family feeling 'unknowing'. People have great difficulty assimilating information pertaining to uncertainty and featuring threat, even when the threat is psychosocial or perceived. Many families will have listened to, and acknowledged, information that they have then not retained. The paediatrician, parent and young person may not have appreciated the limited knowledge until this point, not having found the opportunity in regular clinic time to re-ask questions or assess awareness. Furthermore, a young woman transferring to PAG from paediatrics may have been 'protected' by parents and occasionally health care professionals from potentially upsetting or confusing self-knowledge.

Sensitive support of a young person towards full knowledge of their body and its full potential takes time. Often a psychologist can lead this process with the help of the gynaecologist and, ideally, a specialist nurse. The clinical tool 'The Story of Sex Development' – free to download at www.dsdfamilies .org – provides a way to map sex development for anyone. Rather than taking a normative position that privileges 'typical' or 'normal' development ('this is normal – then this is you'), the template maps any and all development and tracks the implications for variations in sex characteristics. See Figure 14.3.

Making individualised notes on printed materials for people to take away prompts information rehearsal and retention. With encouragement, acceptance and a sense of fun the young person could explain to their partner, parent or friend how the template works. Any discussion that can elicit comment, reflection or questions is a good one. We are aware that during uncomfortable conversations patients will often smile and agree, say they have

understood, and that they are happy with what they have been told, treatment to date and plans for the future. This is particularly challenging when parents offer this 'disguised compliance' in relation to information-sharing with their child. Follow-up on a patient's concordance or understanding of self-management needs, long-term implications of diagnosis and so on can be shared with other team members.

14.10 Rare Diagnoses: Everything Has Changed, and Everything Remains the Same

When a girl is referred with primary amenorrhea, she and her parents will be hoping that the gynaecologist will quickly work out what small matter has caused this glitch and remedy it, quite possibly or even preferably with an operation. If investigations reveal that the girl has XY DSD such as a gonadal dysgenesis (Swyer syndrome), 17 beta-hydroxylase deficiency syndrome or androgen insensitivity syndrome, the young person and her family must begin a journey of understanding. Future expectations, taken for granted and perhaps not really thought about yet, may become the focus of intense loss. And yet, the patient is healthy and physically exactly the same person she was before she learned this surprising information about her body.

We know that it is difficult to retain information when receiving a threatening diagnosis [14]. However, when patients need to travel a great distance to a specialist service there is a pressure to avoid a series of short appointments and instead establish a coherent narrative. Extended appointments with different sections or breaks can involve different professionals with overlapping information exchanges including re-telling diagnostic information, summaries, questions, standard written material and bespoke take-home information. When giving complex or highly impactful information to a patient in a PAG service it is helpful for the patient to have a family member with her. Wherever possible, the PAG psychologist should be part of the consultation too: observing patient – parent responses, tracking understanding and bringing information about psychological acceptance. It can be helpful for the psychologist or nurse to make notes for the patient to take away. The psychologist can provide follow-up appointments to enable the patient to reflect upon and assimilate

Bringing it all together

On this page we bring together all we have learned in 10 steps about typical and less typical sex development.

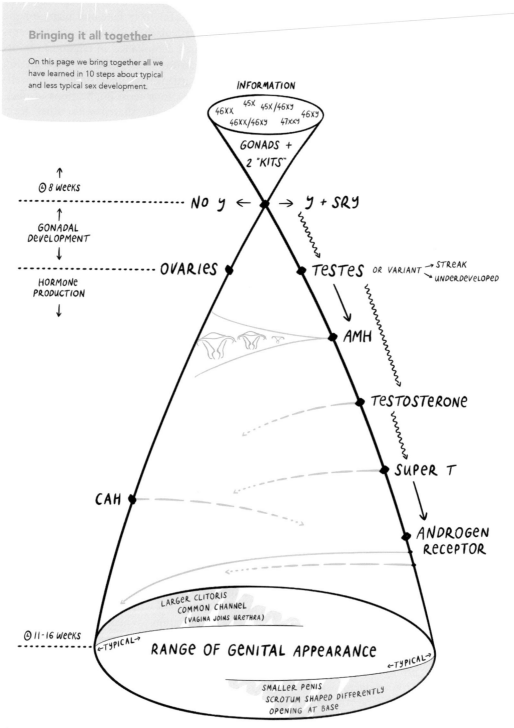

Figure 14.3 A map for everyone's sex development from *The Story of Sex Development* by dsdfamilies. Reproduced with permission from dsdfamilies and Emily Tulloh, illustrator.

Box 14.7 Am I Normal?

PAG services are presented with challenges that are characteristically psychological or social in nature, such as requests for cosmetic genital surgery. A PAG service must use training focussed on social and clinical psychology, then continually develop their practice and maintain their team approach in response to varied, often distressing presentations and challenging consultations.

'Female sexual response involves mind-emotion-body interactions about which researchers and surgeons still know very little, and which are usually beyond the conscious control of the woman. In the supposed cause of improving women's sexual function by making them feel better, surgeons are scarring and destroying sexually responsive tissue' [15, p. 87].

the new information within their existing values and ways of thinking.

A person who has lived a female role throughout childhood and has anticipated her future woman-hood will be surprised to be told that she has XY chromosomes, internal testes, no womb and limited vaginal depth beyond a 'dimple' opening. A common reaction is for shock to arrest her flexible thinking, with the young woman and her parents reaching out to have the 'previous position' 'restored' (e.g. calls for action and request for rapid gonadectomy, dilation, surgery and lifelong HRT). Without psychological containment to promote consideration of possible futures based on preferences, derived from careful reflection upon individual values, we perpetuate poor clinical practice of the past. It is not enough to provide 'time to think' based on the time between consultations. The person and family need support and scaffolding to gain pertinent information and consider its implications in their specific case. Previous cohorts of patients report cosmetic genital surgeries without fully considered consent, gonadectomy without the level of understanding to enable full consent or appreciation of the risks and consequential need for engagement with ongoing care. Many individuals and groups have used social media platforms to raise awareness of past care that did not provide information, time and assistance to consider body image, gender identity, sexuality, possible parenthood, and sexual function

beyond vaginal penetration. Many voices say that their psychological care was inadequate or absent. Conversely, some argue that it is over-pathologising to be asked to see a psychological professional as part of physical care. They may seek opportunities to reflect and make 'treatment' decisions assisted by peers and non-professional information and support organisations. However, demonstrating an understanding and actively engaging in health care discussions must be a prerequisite of irreversible medical or surgical interventions. It is the responsibility of the PAG service to go beyond the principles of informed consent or legal requirement. A table of professional behaviours to facilitate informed consent is published to guide practitioners [2].

14.11 Peer Information and Support

A common but regretful comment from many women with rare diagnoses such as androgen insensitivity syndrome (AIS), or even the more common congenital adrenal hyperplasia (CAH), is that they have never met anyone with the same condition. While introducing patients to each other can raise governance challenges when it is choreographed by health care professionals, directing people to peer organisations puts the individual in control. Referring to support groups can be made more difficult by factors such as the names of organisations, or by the terms they use being disfavoured by the people they aim to support or speak on behalf of. People active in creating peer opportunities or organisations may be inured to certain language or in other cases have reclaimed language once thought of within medical professions as pejorative, inaccurate or inappropriate. This was seen in the 1990s with the Hermaphrodites with Attitude group and currently with organisations using the terms *dsd* and *intersex*. However, the benefits of meeting others who have experience and knowledge to share outweighs the clinician's discomfort with explaining terms or language that might feel out of place in a medical setting. How, in the pursuit of open, honest acceptance, can we readily say 'gonad', 'phallus' and 'clitoris' to a PAG patient but then struggle to explain terms they may encounter such as different sex development or intersex?

Services often aspire to run local information events where people with similar diagnoses or demands of treatment can learn together. Design of events should be led by people who are the target attenders to improve the acceptability and, hopefully, uptake. Matters such as range and depth of topic along with practical details such as venue, times and refreshments should be co-designed in every instance.

14.12 Meeting the Challenge of Culturally Sensitive PAG Care

When health care centralises understanding over technological interventions and normative treatments it is more likely to be sensitive to a patient's culture. Basing care on the patient's values and broad goals can further safeguard against clashes between a patient's culture and any treatment offered. Exploring a patient's cultural socialisation and personal values as part of care planning and decision-making can lead to rich discussion, promote understanding and hopefully prevent dissatisfaction. However, in PAG care there may be instances where patient values and hopes for intervention may be in conflict with the treatments offered, particularly if hetero-normative pressures on the patient are high. As health workers we should seek support from colleagues when this happens. Offering patients peer support opportunities designed for specific communities can be an extremely powerful if adequate engagement efforts are possible.

Key Learning Points

- Psychological care in PAG is preventative in focus.
- Keep flexible adult futures in mind – treatments have permanent effects.
- Update to non-normative language and update patients.
- Look for meaning in distress or troubled behaviour.
- Peer contact and information can be transformative for many.

References

1. British Psychological Society. Response to the American Psychiatric Association: DSM-5 development. 2011. https://dxrevisionwatch .files.wordpress.com/2012/02/dsm-5-2011-bps-response.pdf.

2. Chadwick PM, Tamar-Mattis J, Liao L-M. Obtaining informed consent in pediatric and adolescent gynaecology practice: from ethical principles to ethical behaviours. In: Creighton S, Balen A, Breech L, Liao L-M, editors. Pediatric and adolescent gynaecology: a problem-based approach. Cambridge: Cambridge University Press; 2018. p. 45–52.

3. Liao L-M, Roen K. The role of psychologists in multi-disciplinary teams for intersex/diverse sex development: interviews with British and Swedish clinical specialists. Psychol Sexual. 2021;12(3):202–16.

4. Maslach C, Leiter MP. Early predictors of job burnout and engagement. J Appl Psychiatr. 2008;93 (3):498–512.

5. West CP, Huschka MM, Novotny PJ, Sloan JA, Kolars JC, Hanermann TM, et al. Association of perceived medical errors with resident distress and empathy: a prospective longitudinal study. JAMA. 2006;296(9):1071–8.

6. Gilbert P. The compassionate mind. London: Robinson; 2013.

7. Trzeciak S, Roberts BW, Mazzarelli AJ. Compassionomics: hypothesis and experimental approach. Med Hypotheses. 2017;107:92–7.

8. Trzeciak S, Mazzarelli A. Campassionomics: the revolutionary scientific evidence that caring makes a difference. Pensacola, FL: Studer Group; 2019.

9. Davison SN. Facilitating advance care planning for patients with end-stage renal disease: the patient perspective. Clin J Am Soc Nephrol. 2006;1 (5):1023–8.

10. Hack TF, Denger L, Parker P. The communication goals and needs of cancer patients: a review. Psycho-oncology. 2005;14:831–45.

11. Alderson J, Magritte E, Tulloh E. Top tips for talking about differences of sex development. 2018. www .dsdfamilies.org/parents/talking.

12. Pasterski V, Mastroyannopoulou K, Wright D, Zucker KJ, Hughes IA. Predictors of posttraumatic stress in parents of children diagnosed with a disorder of sex development. Arch Sex Behav. 2014;43(2):369–75.

13. Johnstone L, Boyle M, Cromby J, Dillon J, Harper D, Kinderman P, et al. The Power Threat Meaning Framework: towards the identification of patterns in emotional distress, unusual experiences and troubled or troubling behaviour, as an alternative to functional psychiatric diagnosis. Leicester, UK: British Psychological Society; 2018.

14. Ley P. Memory for medical information. Br J Soc Clin Psychol. 1979;18(2):245–55.

15. Cook H. A historical analysis of beliefs supporting female genital cosmetic surgery. In: Creighton S, Liao L-M, editors. Female genital cosmetic surgery: solution to what problem? Cambridge: Cambridge University Press; 2019. p. 80–89.

Legal and Ethical Aspects of Paediatric and Adolescent Gynaecology

Parivakkam S. Arunakumari

15.1 Introduction

As a specialty, paediatric and adolescent gynaecology (PAG) is relatively young. However, the legal and ethical principles underpinning its practice are ancient, dating back to Hippocratic times. This chapter covers only the legal and ethical aspects of PAG outlined in the RCOG ATSM curriculum – consent and confidentiality, child maltreatment, safeguarding and female genital mutilation (FGM).

15.2 Consent and Confidentiality

15.2.1 Consent

15.2.1.1 Introduction

Good medical practice states that doctors must safeguard and protect the health and well-being of children and young people. Well-being includes treating them as individuals and respecting their views, as well as considering their physical and emotional welfare [1]. Respecting their views implies imparting information to involve them in decision-making.

15.2.1.2 Sexual Activity, Consent and the Law

In law, any competent young person in the United Kingdom can consent to medical treatment, including contraception. Young people aged 16 years of age and older, including those with a disability/impairment, are presumed to be competent to give consent to medical treatment unless otherwise demonstrated. For young people under the age of 16 years, however, competence to consent has to be demonstrated [2].

The age of consent to sexual activity in the United Kingdom is 16 years [2]. Although unlawful, mutually agreed sexual activity between under-16-year-olds of similar age would not generally lead to prosecution unless there was evidence of abuse or exploitation. Under the Sexual Offences Act 2003, a girl under 13

years of age is not considered capable of giving her consent to sexual intercourse [3]. According to the Sexual Offences Act of 2009, sexual activity with a male or female aged under 13 years will be 'rape of a young child' [2].

15.2.1.3 Assessing Competence

Competence is demonstrated if the young person is able to

1. Understand the treatment, its purpose and nature and why it is being proposed
2. Understand its benefits, risks and alternatives
3. Understand in broader terms what the consequences of the treatment will be
4. Retain the information for long enough to use it and weigh up in order to arrive at a decision [2]

Children under the age of 16 can consent to their own treatment if they're believed to have enough intelligence, competence and understanding to fully appreciate what is involved in their treatment. This is known as being Gillick competent.

15.2.1.4 Capacity to Consent

The working test for assessing capacity in young people is the same as that for adults. Only if the young person is able to understand, retain, use and weigh the information, and communicate their decision to others can they consent to the treatment [1]. The assessment of a young person's capacity to make a decision about contraception or medical treatment is a matter of clinical judgement guided by professional practice and legal requirements. Assumptions should not be made about an individual's capacity to consent based on age alone or on disability [2].

15.2.1.5 Fraser Guidelines

It is considered good practice to follow the Fraser guidelines in providing contraceptive advice to young people under the age of 16 years without parental consent [2]. The Fraser criteria include the following:

1. The young person understands the professional's advice.
2. The young person cannot be persuaded to inform their parents.
3. The young person is likely to begin, or continue having, sexual intercourse with or without contraceptive treatment.
4. The young person's physical or mental health, or both, is likely to suffer unless the young person receives contraceptive advice and/or treatment.
5. The young person's best interests require them to receive contraceptive advice and/or treatment with or without parental consent.

15.2.1.6 Young People with Capacity: Refusal of Treatment

By virtue of the Family Reform Act 1969, people aged 16–17 years are presumed to be capable of consenting to their own medical treatment and any ancillary procedures, including anaesthesia. However, unlike the case with adults, the refusal of a competent person aged 16–17 years may, in certain circumstances, be overridden by a person with parental responsibility or by a court [3].

It should be noted that 'parents cannot override the competent consent of a young person to treatment that is considered to be in the best interest of the young person'. In England, Wales and Northern Ireland, the law on parents overriding young people's competent refusal is complex [1]. Resort to the courts is advised.

15.2.1.7 Young People without Capacity

Where a child lacks the capacity to consent, only a holder of 'parental responsibility' or the court can give consent to treatment on behalf of a minor [3]. It is usually sufficient to have consent from one parent. If parents cannot agree and disputes cannot be resolved informally, legal advice should be sought [1].

The legal framework for the treatment of young people aged 16–17 years who lack capacity to consent differs across the United Kingdom. Refer to the GMC guidance for further details [1].

15.2.2 Confidentiality

15.2.2.1 Significance

A confidential sexual health service is essential for the welfare of children and young people. Concern about

confidentiality is the biggest deterrent to young people asking for sexual health advice. The same duties of confidentiality apply when using, sharing or disclosing information about children and young people as about adults [1].

15.2.2.2 Disclosure

However, this duty of confidentiality is not absolute. Disclosure of relevant information with appropriate people or agencies is usually necessary under the following conditions:

1. Where sexual activity involves children under 13, who are considered in law unable to consent
2. If the child or young person is involved in abusive or seriously harmful sexual activity, including that which involves

   - A young person too immature to understand or consent
   - Big differences in age, maturity or power between sexual partners
   - A young person's sexual partner having a position of trust
   - Force or the threat of force, emotional or psychological pressure, bribery or payment, either to engage in sexual activity or to keep it secret
   - Drugs or alcohol used to influence a young person to engage in sexual activity when they otherwise would not
   - A person known to the police or child protection agencies as having had abusive relationships with children or young people [1]

15.2.2.3 Disclosure without Consent

Consent of the young person must be sought in the first instance if they have the capacity to consent, unless it is deemed inappropriate or impractical to ask for consent. Inform the child or young person the reason for the disclosure, the information that will be shared and with whom, and ask for consent for the disclosure. However, consent is not essential

1. If there is an overriding public interest in the disclosure
2. When the disclosure is required by law
3. When the disclosure is in the best interests of the child [1]

If the child or the young person refuses consent, or if it is not practical or appropriate to ask for consent, disclosure may still be necessary to protect the child or young person, or someone else, from risk of death or serious harm. Such cases may arise, for example, if

1. A child or young person is at risk of neglect or of sexual, physical or emotional abuse
2. The information would help in the prevention, detection or prosecution of serious crime, usually crime against the person
3. A child or young person is involved in behaviour that might put them or others at risk of serious harm, such as serious addiction, self-harm or joyriding [1]

15.2.2.4 Caldicott Principles

Patient information is generally held under legal and ethical obligations of confidentiality [4]. The Caldicott principles include the following:

1. Justify the purpose of using, sharing or disclosing patient-identifiable information (PII).
2. Don't use PII unless it is absolutely necessary.
3. Use the minimum necessary PII.
4. Access to PII should be on a strict need-to-know basis.
5. All staff should be aware of their responsibilities.
6. All staff should understand and comply with the law.
7. The duty to share information can be as important as the duty to protect confidentiality [4].

15.3 Child Maltreatment

15.3.1 Introduction

Child maltreatment is recognised as a significant public health concern globally with serious lifelong consequences. It is morally reprehensible, yet ordinarily prevalent in all sections of society.

15.3.2 Definitions

15.3.2.1 Child Maltreatment

All forms of physical and/or emotional ill treatment, sexual abuse, neglect or negligent treatment or commercial or other exploitation, resulting in actual or potential harm to the child's health, survival, development or dignity in the context of a relationship of responsibility, trust or power [5].

15.3.2.2 Children

Anyone who has not yet reached their eighteenth birthday is a child. The fact that a child has reached 16 years of age, is living independently or is in further education, is a member of the armed forces, is in hospital or is in custody in the secure estate does not change their entitlements to services or protection [6].

15.3.3 Scale of the Problem

Following several high-profile media cases starting from Maria Cowell (1973) to Victoria Climbie (2000) and Peter Connelly (Baby P 2007), there has been an increase in child protection activity in the United Kingdom. The number of children on child protection plans has increased from 26,400 in 2006 to 42,900 in 2012 and 57,000 in 2015 [7].

Every year, 40,000 children under 15 years of age are victims of homicide.

15.3.4 Significance

Child maltreatment has devastatingly disastrous short-term and long-term repercussions on the victim, the family and the society at large.

Short-Term Consequences
- Unintended pregnancy
- Sexually transmitted infections
- Physical trauma – fractures, bruises, lacerations, burns, abusive head trauma
- Death, disability

Long-Term Consequences
- Behavioural: smoking, drug abuse, alcohol misuse
- Psychological: anxiety, depression, post-traumatic stress disorder, suicide
- Social: difficulty in sustaining long-term relationships, poor parenting skills
- Economic: difficulty in getting and holding jobs
- Academic: poor academic achievement, lack of qualifications
- Criminal: perpetuating and being a victim of crime, antisocial behaviour and violence
- Chronic disease: heart disease, cancer, hypertension [8]

15.3.5 Risk Factors for Child Maltreatment

Knowledge of risk factors aids in the early recognition of all types of child maltreatment.

Parent Factors
- Alcohol dependence
- Substance misuse

- Mental health issues
- Chronic ill health
- Learning difficulties
- Emotional volatility
- Unemployed or lack of financial support
- Engaged in criminal activity
- History of abuse as a child

Child Factors

- Special-needs child
- Learning disabilities
- Mental health problems
- Abnormal physical features
- Result of an unwanted pregnancy
- Prematurity

Relationship Factors

- Poor parent–child bonding
- Intimate partner violence
- Parent is socially isolated
- Parent does not have the support of extended family
- Family breakdown

Community Factors

- Poverty
- Lack of housing
- Lack of educational opportunities
- Member of a gang
- Lack of support services for families in need
- High tolerance for violence [6]

Societal Factors

- Without adequate legislation against child maltreatment
- Cultural norms that glorify or promote violence
- Social, economic and health policies that lead to poor living standards or socioeconomic inequality [7,8]

15.3.6 Classification of Child Maltreatment

The WHO classifies child maltreatment into four main categories:

- Physical abuse
- Emotional abuse
- Sexual abuse
- Neglect

The United Kingdom recognises child sexual exploitation as a fifth category [6].

15.3.7 Physical Abuse

15.3.7.1 Definition

Physical abuse is a form of abuse that may involve hitting, shaking, throwing, poisoning, burning, scalding, drowning, suffocating or otherwise causing physical harm to a child or failing to protect a child from that harm.

15.3.7.2 Recognising Physical Abuse

It is important to remember at the outset that injuries are quite common in school-age children and may have explanations other than child abuse.

Physical Indicators

- Injury in a non-ambulant child
- Unexplained bruises or burns, particularly if they are recurrent
- Human bite marks, welts or bald spots
- Untreated injuries
- Unexplained lacerations, abrasions or fractures

Behavioural Indicators

- Deliberate self-harm
- Chronic runaway
- Improbable excuses given to explain injuries
- Aggressive or withdrawn
- Fear of returning home
- Reluctant to have physical contact
- Clothing inappropriate to weather – worn to hide part of body [9,10]

Factors That Heighten the Suspicion of Maltreatment

1. Unclear mechanism of injury
2. Discrepancy in history between carers or between carers and child
3. Inconsistent story
4. Child gives impression of being coached
5. Delayed presentation
6. Abnormal carer–child interaction
7. Unusual location of injury, e.g. behind ears or on upper thighs [7]

15.3.8 Fabricated Illness

Physical harm may be caused when a parent or carer fabricates the symptoms of, or deliberately induces, illness in a child.

Suspect induced illness if a child's history, presentations or findings of assessments, examinations or investigations lead to a discrepancy with a recognised clinical picture and one or more of the following is present:

- Reported symptoms appear only when the carer is present.
- An inexplicably poor response is seen to prescribed medication or other treatment.
- New symptoms are reported as soon as previous ones have resolved.
- The history of events is biologically unlikely.
- Multiple opinions are sought and disputed by the carer.
- The child's normal daily activities are being compromised [9].

15.3.9 Neglect

15.3.9.1 Definition

Neglect is the persistent failure to meet a child's basic physical and/or psychological needs, likely to result in the serious impairment of the child's health or development [6].

15.3.9.2 Types

Neglect can take various forms, including the following:

- Medical: missed clinic appointments, non-compliance with medical recommendations, poor dentition, failure to engage with child health promotion programmes such as immunisation or screening
- Nutritional: inadequate growth, stunted development, severe obesity
- Educational: poor school attendance, truanting
- Failure to provide supervision: recurrent accidents, sexual exploitation
- Abandonment: child found unattended in home, missing from home, run away [7]

15.3.9.3 Recognising Emotional Abuse

Physical Indicators

- Constant hunger
- Poor personal hygiene – dirty or smelly, especially if ingrained
- Poor/inappropriate state of clothing/footwear
- Untreated medical problems
- Severe persistent infections – scabies, head lice
- Emaciation
- Constant tiredness
- Flinching when approached or touched

Behavioural Indicators

- Tiredness, listlessness
- Compulsive stealing, begging or scavenging
- Low self-esteem
- Frequently absent or late
- Lack of social relationships [9,10]

15.3.10 Emotional Abuse

15.3.10.1 Definition

Emotional abuse is the persistent emotional maltreatment of a child such as to cause severe and persistent adverse effects on the child's emotional development.

It may involve conveying to a child that they are worthless or unloved, inadequate or valued only insofar as they meet the needs of another person. It may include not giving the child opportunities to express their views, deliberately silencing them or 'making fun' of what they say or how they communicate. It may feature age- or developmentally inappropriate expectations being imposed on children. These may include interactions that are beyond a child's developmental capability, as well as overprotection and limitation of exploration and learning or preventing the child from participating in normal social interactions. It may involve seeing or hearing the ill treatment of another. It may involve serious bullying (including cyberbullying) causing children to feel frightened or in danger or the exploitation or the corruption of children. Some level of emotional abuse is involved in all types of maltreatment of a child, though it may occur alone [6].

15.3.10.2 Recognising Emotional Abuse

Physical Indicators

- Sudden speech disorders
- Wetting/soiling
- Signs of solvent abuse – mouth sores, smells of glue
- Neurotic behaviours – thumb sucking, hair twisting, rocking

Behavioural Indicators in the Child

- Fearful, withdrawn
- Low self-esteem
- Aggressive towards others or oppositional
- Poor social skills

- Inappropriate emotional responses to situations – inconsolable crying, temper tantrums
- Indiscriminate contact or affection seeking
- Over-friendliness to strangers, including health care professionals
- Excessive clinginess
- Persistently resorting to gaining attention
- Demonstrating excessively 'good' behaviour to prevent parental or carer disapproval
- Failing to seek or accept appropriate comfort or affection from an appropriate person when significantly distressed
- Coercive controlling behaviour towards parents or carers
- Lack of ability to understand and recognise emotions [9,10]

Behavioural Indicators in the Adolescent
- Risk-taking behaviours – often excessive
- Frequent rages on minor provocations
- Few, if any, friends
- Unexpected manner and language for age
- Interpersonal behaviour towards parent/carer showing
  - Dislike or lack of cooperation
  - Lack of interest or low responsiveness
  - High levels of anger or annoyance
  - Passive or withdrawn behaviours

Behavioural Indicators in the Parent/Carer
- Negativity or hostility towards a child or young person
- Rejection or scapegoating of a child or young person
- Developmentally inappropriate expectations of or interactions with a child, including inappropriate threats or methods of disciplining
- Exposure to frightening or traumatic experiences
- Using the child for the fulfilment of the adult's needs (e.g. in marital disputes)
- Failure to promote the child's appropriate socialisation (e.g. involving children in unlawful activities, isolation, not providing stimulation or education)
- Refusal to allow a child or young person to speak to a practitioner on their own when it is necessary for the assessment of the child or young person [9,10]

15.3.11 Child Sexual Abuse

15.3.11.1 Definition
Child sexual abuse involves forcing or enticing a child or young person to take part in sexual activities, not necessarily involving a high level of violence, whether or not the child is aware of what is happening. The activities may involve physical contact, including assault by penetration (e.g. rape or oral sex) or non-penetrative acts, such as masturbation, kissing, rubbing and touching outside of clothing. They may also include non-contact activities, such as involving children in looking at or producing, sexual images, watching sexual activities, encouraging children to behave in sexually inappropriate ways or grooming a child in preparation for abuse. Sexual abuse can take place online, and technology can be used to facilitate offline abuse. Sexual abuse is not perpetrated solely by adult males. Women can also commit acts of sexual abuse, as can other children [6].

15.3.11.2 Recognising CSA
Physical Indicators
- Anal or vaginal soreness or itching
- Genital bruising, erythema, oedema, abrasions or lacerations
- Genital bleeding
- Physical symptoms – pelvic pain, enuresis
- Discomfort when walking or sitting down
- STI – chlamydia, gonorrhoea, herpes, syphilis, trichomonas, HIV
- Pregnancy

Behavioural Indicators
- Sexual behaviour that is indiscriminate, precocious or coercive
- Sexual talk associated with knowledge
- Emulating sexual activity with another child

15.3.12 Child Sexual Exploitation

15.3.12.1 Definition
Child sexual exploitation (CSE) is a form of a child sexual abuse. It occurs when an individual or group takes advantage of an imbalance of power to coerce, manipulate or deceive a child or young person under the age of 18 into sexual activity (1) in exchange for something the victim needs or wants and/or (2) for the financial advantage or increased status of the

perpetrator or facilitator. The victim may have been sexually exploited even if the sexual activity appears consensual. CSE does not always involve physical contact; it can also occur through the use of technology [6].

15.3.12.2 Recognising CSE

Alerting features in the history include the following:

- Young person going missing from home, care or education
- Going missing overnight or arriving home late
- Losing contact with peers and hanging out with older age groups or antisocial groups
- Possessing expensive items – such as mobile phones, branded accessories – which they can't explain
- Excessive and secret use of the internet and social media
- Spending time in places of concern – brothels, hotels [9,10]

15.4 Safeguarding

15.4.1 Rights of the Child

The UN Convention on the Rights of the Child 1989 is an international agreement setting out the rights of every child:

- Survival rights: The child's right to life and to the most basic needs – food, shelter and access to health care
- Developmental rights: To achieve their full potential – education, play, freedom of thought, conscience and religion; those with disabilities to receive special services
- Protection rights: Against all forms of abuse, neglect, exploitation and discrimination
- Participation rights: To take an active role in their communities and nations

Under this convention, governments are legally obliged to meet children's basic needs and help them reach their full potential. In the United Kingdom, the statutory framework is laid out in the DOH publication [6].

15.4.2 Definitions

Safeguarding is defined as

- Protecting children from maltreatment
- Preventing impairment of children's health or development

- Ensuring that children are growing up in circumstances consistent with the provision of safe and effective care
- Taking action to enable all children to have the best outcomes [6]

Child protection is part of safeguarding and promoting welfare. This refers to the activity that is undertaken to meet the statutory obligations to protect specific children who are suffering, or are likely to suffer, significant harm [6].

15.4.3 Statutory Responsibilities

The high cost of abuse (acts of commission) and neglect (acts of omission) to individuals and society underpins the duty on all agencies to be proactive in safeguarding children. Core Services National Service Framework for Children, Young People and Maternity Services 2004, Department of Health, www.assets.publishing.service.gov.uk [7]

Safeguarding and child protection are closely interlinked and are statutory duties of all health care professionals. It should not be forgotten that cruelty to children and young people is a criminal offence.

A safeguarding partner in relation to a local authority area in England is defined under the Children Act 2004 as

1. The local authority
2. A Clinical Commissioning Group for an area, any part of which falls within the local authority area and
3. The Chief Officer of Police for an area, any part of which falls within the local authority area

The three safeguarding partners should agree on ways to coordinate their safeguarding services; act as a strategic leadership group; and implement local and national learning, including from serious child safeguarding incidents [6].

Child protection is the responsibility of all doctors. Yet it is challenging in clinical practice, as

- It goes against the assumption that parents usually have their children's best interests at heart
- It can involve confronting carers/parents who may be manipulative or aggressive
- It requires a detailed and thorough evaluation of the history and examination to identify inconsistencies and interpret subtle findings, as the issues are often complex
- It depends on genuinely good multi-professional teamwork and respect of colleagues [12]

15.4.4 General Principles of Management

The challenge will be in identifying the abuse and responding proportionately in a manner that safeguards the child and other children in the family, whilst at the same time offering the family support, guidance and respect.

For the broad principles of working with children, young people, parents and carers, please refer to NICE NG76.

15.4.4.1 Assessing Risk

- History: This begins with a detailed history, being cognizant of the alerting features in the history. It is important to create an opportunity to speak to the child/young person alone.
- Examination: Clear, concise and contemporaneous documentation is vital. It is important to distinguish between observations and interpretations.
- Communicating risk: If there is any suspicion of maltreatment, refer to the professional with expertise in child protection. All gynaecologists should have a clear idea of how, when and why to refer to local child protection specialists in the Trust.

It is vital that all doctors have the confidence to act if they believe that a child or young person may be being abused or neglected. Taking action will be justified, even if it turns out that the child or the young person is not at risk of, or suffering, abuse or neglect, as long as the concerns are honestly held and reasonable and the doctor takes action through appropriate channels, sharing only the relevant information. In sharing concerns about possible abuse or neglect, the health professional is not making the final decision about how best to protect the child or the young person. That is the role of the local authority children's services and, ultimately, the courts [13].

Collaborative work across the health sector, as well as across educational, social care and justice organisations, is imperative. The 5P approach to support multiagency working includes the following:

- Physical systems – IT or paper based
- People – for joined-up working
- Policies
- Protocols
- Pathways – to promote responsibility and accountability [14]

15.4.4.2 Summary

All staff working with young people should know

- How to access national and local child protection guidance and procedures
- Who provides advice and expertise locally within their service
- Under what circumstances child protection procedures should be initiated
- What services are available locally, when and how to refer
- How child protection procedures may affect different groups

15.4.5 Relevant Guidance

15.4.5.1 Laming Report

Lord Laming submitted his report on the inquiry into the murder of child abuse victim Victoria Climbie in 2003. The report contained 108 recommendations under four captions – general, social care, health care and police – of which 64–90 pertained to health care. He subsequently published a progress report titled 'The Protection of Children in England' in 2009. This made 58 recommendations, all of which were accepted by the government.

15.4.5.2 GMC Guidance

- Good Medical Practice
- 0–18 years: Guidance for all doctors
- Confidentiality: good practice in handling patient information
- Consent: patients and doctors making decisions together

15.5 Female Genital Mutilation (FGM)

15.5.1 Definition

The World Health Organization (WHO) defines FGM as 'all procedures involving partial or total removal of the external female genitalia or other injury to the female genital organs for non-medical reasons' [15]. FGM is practised in 28 African countries, the Middle East, Indonesia and Malaysia but does not appear to be as prevalent in migrant families in the United Kingdom.

Reasons given by practitioners for the performance of FGM may include reduction of libido, means of ensuring chastity, preparation of a girl for marriage and misinformation as a necessary religious practice by misinterpretation of scriptures [8].

15.5.2 Significance

FGM has no health benefits. WHO and the International Federation of Gynecology and Obstetrics (FIOG) have openly condemned FGM. FGM is a human rights violation and a form of child abuse, breaching the UN Convention on the Rights of the Child, and is a severe form of violence against women and girls.

15.5.3 WHO FGM Classification

Type 1, Partial or total removal of the clitoris and/or the prepuce (clitoridectomy)

Type 2. Partial or total removal of the clitoris and the labia minora, with or without excision of the labia majora (excision)

Type 3. Narrowing of the vaginal orifice with creation of a covering seal by cutting and appositioning the labia minora and/or the labia majora, with or without excision of the clitoris (infibulation)

Type 4. All other harmful procedures to the female genitalia for non-medical purposes, for example pricking, piercing, incising, scraping and cauterisation

15.5.4 Presentation

FGM is often an incidental finding in an adolescent during a consultation for contraceptive advice, assessment of menstrual dysfunction, genital examination or during the performance of TOP.

15.5.5 FGM and UK Law

All health professionals must be aware that

- FGM is illegal unless it is a surgical operation on a girl or woman irrespective of her age
  - ○ Which is necessary for her physical or mental health or
  - ○ She is in any stage of labour, or has just given birth, for purposes connected with the labour or birth.
- It is illegal to arrange, or assist in arranging, for a UK national or UK resident to be taken overseas for the purpose of FGM.
- It is an offence for those with parental responsibility to fail to protect a girl from the risk

of FGM, even if the parents themselves did not perform the procedure.

The two Acts on FGM (FGM Act 2003 and FGM (Scotland) Act 2005) make it an offence for any person

- To excise, infibulate or otherwise mutilate the whole or any part of a person's labia majora, labia minora or clitoris, or
- To aid, abet, counsel or procure the performance by another person of any of those acts on that other person's own body, or
- To aid, abet, counsel or procure a person to excise, infibulate or otherwise mutilate the whole or any part of her own labia majora, labia minora or clitoris.
- Serious Crime Act 2015 made amendments to the FGM Act, which are
  1. Mandatory reporting for all under-18s
  2. FGM Protection Orders for girls at risk
  3. Lifelong anonymity for victims of FGM
  4. Extra-territorial jurisdiction over offences of FGM committed abroad by UK nationals

15.5.6 Legal and Regulatory Responsibilities of Health Care Professionals

15.5.6.1 Data Recording

- Data recording is mandatory for all women identified as having FGM.
- Document FGM diagnoses in medical records (even if FGM is not the reason for presentation).
- If genital examination is performed and the type of FGM is identified, record FGM type as per WHO classifications.
- Document further details in accordance with the HSCIC FGM Enhanced Dataset.
- Explain to the woman that her personal data will be transmitted to the HSCIC for the purpose of FGM prevalence monitoring and that the data will not be anonymised.

15.5.6.2 Mandatory Reporting

15.5.6.2.1 Children under 18 Years

If FGM is confirmed (on examination or if the patient or parent says it has been done), refer as a matter of urgency to the police and social services. This should be done within 1 month of confirmation but ideally before end of play of the next working day.

If FGM is suspected (but not confirmed) or the girl is at risk (but has not had FGM), refer to social services. The urgency of the referral depends on the degree of risk.

15.5.6.2.2 Non-pregnant Women with FGM

There is no requirement to report unless a related child is at risk. The patient's right to confidentiality must be respected if they do not wish any action to be taken. No reports to the police or social care should be made in these cases [5]. The FGM should still be recorded in accordance with the HSCIC Enhanced Dataset.

15.5.7 Legal Management

When a woman with FGM is identified, the health professional must explain the UK law on FGM. The health professional must understand the difference between recording (documenting FGM in the medical records for data collection) and reporting (making a referral to police and/or social services) and their responsibilities with regard to these.

The health professional must be familiar with the requirements of the HSCIC FGM Enhanced Dataset and explain its purpose to the woman. The requirement for her personal data to be submitted without anonymisation to the HSCIC, in order to prevent duplication of data, should be explained. However, she should also be told that all personal data are anonymised at the point of statistical analysis and publication.

The requirement to report (making a referral to the police or social services) depends on whether an adult or child is affected. In accordance with Children's Act 1989, any child with confirmed or suspected FGM, or a child considered to be at risk of FGM, must be reported, if necessary without the consent of the parents. Information should also be shared with the GP and health visitor.

All health care professionals working with children must be advocates against FGM and supportive of legislation to end this practice.

15.5.8 Female Genital Cosmetic Surgery

FGCS refers to non-medically indicated cosmetic surgical procedures which change the structure and appearance of the healthy external genitalia of women, or internally in the case of vaginal tightening. This definition includes the most common procedure,

labiaplasty, as well as others, such as hymenoplasty, vaginal reconstruction and vaginal rejuvenation [16].

In a consideration of the question 'Should FGCS be regarded ethically and legally as FGM?' Kelly and Foster note, 'Professional opinion on FGCS is changing. Internationally, a number of OG colleges expressly disapprove FGCS, being concerned about the motivation of women seeking surgery, the efficacy, safety of these procedures, and the potential to further traumatise patients who are anxious or insecure about their genital appearance and/or sexual function. In general FGCS should not be undertaken in the NHS, unless it is medically indicated' [17].

> There is no scientific evidence to support the practice of labiaplasty, and in girls under the age of 18, the risk of harm is even more significant. In the absence of an identifiable disease and until the evidence demonstrates to the contrary, labiaplasty should not be performed in girls under the age of 18 years. [18]

15.6 Conclusion

It behoves all professionals working with children to be familiar with the legal and ethical principles governing the practice of PAG.

Key Learning Points

- The legal age of consent to medical treatment, including contraception, in the United Kingdom is 16 years. For under-16s, capacity to consent has to be demonstrated.
- Confidentiality is paramount, but not absolute. The duty to share information is as important as the duty to protect information.
- Safeguarding is everyone's responsibility and should be adopted using a child-centred approach.
- All professionals should be alert to the possibility of child maltreatment. If there is any suspicion, refer to professional with expertise in child protection.
- FGM is a criminal offence necessitating reporting to the police and/or social services if confirmed or suspected in children under 18.

References

1. GMC. 0–18 years: guidance for all doctors. 2018.
2. Contraceptive choices for young people. 2019.
3. RCOG. The care of women requesting induced abortion. 2011. www.rcog.org.uk/en/guidelines-

research-services/guidelines/the-care-of-women-requesting-induced-abortion/.

4. Committee FCS. Service standards for sexual and reproductive healthcare. 2015. www.fsrh.org/standards-and-guidance/documents/clinical-standards-service-standards-confidentiality/.

5. Krug EG, Mercy JA, Dahlberg LL, Zwi AB. The world report on violence and health. Lancet. 2002;**360**(9339):1083–8.

6. Her Majesty's Government. Working together to safeguard children: a guide to interagency working to safeguard and promote the welfare of children. 2018.

7. National Service Framework for Children, Young People and Maternity Services for England. Core Services National Service Framework for Children, Young People and Maternity Services 2004, Department of Health, www.assets.publishing.service.gov.uk.

8. Creighton S BA, Breech L, Liao L. Pediatric and adolescent gynecology – a problem based approach. Hoboken, NJ: John Wiley; 2018.

9. WHO. Child maltreatment – infographic. 2017.

10. NICE. Child maltreatment: when to suspect maltreatment in under 18s. 2017.

11. NICE. Child abuse and neglect. 2017.

12. Lissauer TaCW. Illustrated textbook of paediatrics. London: Elsevier; 2018.

13. GMC. Protecting children and young people: the responsibilities of all doctors. 2018.

14. CQC. Not seen, not heard – a review of the arrangements for child safeguarding and healthcare for looked after children in England. 2016.

15. RCOG. Female genital mutilation and its management. 2015. www.rcog.org.uk/en/guidelines-research-services/guidelines/gtg53/.

16. RCOG. Ethical opinion paper – ethical considerations in relation to female genital cosmetic surgery. 2013. www.rcog.org.uk/en/guidelines-research-services/ethics-issues–resources/.

17. RCOG. Ethical Opinion Paper. Ethic considerations in relation to female genital cosmetic surgery (FGCS). 2013. www.rcog.org.uk/globalassets/documents/guidelines/ethics-issues-and-resources/rcog-fgcs-ethical-opinion-paper.pdf.

18. RCOG. Position statement: labial reduction surgery (labiaplasty) on adolescents. 2013. www.rcog.org.uk/globalassets/documents/news/britspag_labiaplasty positionstatement.pdf.

Index